PSYCHIATRY - THEORY, APPLICATIONS AND TREATMENTS

MENTAL HEALTH AND PSYCHIATRY

PSYCHIATRY - THEORY, APPLICATIONS AND TREATMENTS

Additional books in this series can be found on Nova's website under the Series tab.

Additional e-books in this series can be found on Nova's website under the e-book tab.

PSYCHIATRY - THEORY, APPLICATIONS AND TREATMENTS

MENTAL HEALTH AND PSYCHIATRY

ADAM S. WILSON
AND
MICHAEL S. SCHNEIDER
EDITORS

New York

For permission to use material from this book please contact us:
Telephone 631-231-7269; Fax 631-231-8175
Web Site: http://www.novapublishers.com

Library of Congress Cataloging-in-Publication Data

ISBN: 978-1-62417-589-3
Library of Congress Control Number: 2012954738

Published by Nova Science Publishers, Inc. + New York

CONTENTS

PREFACE

In this book, the authors present current research in mental health and psychiatry issues. Topics discussed include the cognitive and emotional processes in approaching personality disorders; sensory impairment and mental health; evidence for epidemiological transition hypothesis for elderly suicides; and the psychiatry of Pellagra.

Chapter 1 – This chapter review the key role played by basic psychological processes in the current conceptualization of personality disorders, the most outstanding models, and the cognitive-behavioral therapies. Currently, there is an increasing tendency towards more dimensional approaches at the expense of more categorical ones. Basic psychological processes are more relevant for dimensional approaches. In this regard, a number of models will be described: the 7 factor model, the Big Five model, the biosocial model, and the cognitive models. Likewise, the basics of both cognitive-behavioral approaches to personality disorders will be outlined. Finally, the role of perception, attention, memory, learning, impulsiveness, emotion, and the way cognitive-behavioral therapies cope with them will also be reviewed. All these processes should be given due relevance.

Chapter 2 – Sensory impairment - hearing impairment, visual impairment or deaf-blindness - is found to increase the risk of developing mental health problems of almost all kinds. The aim of this chapter is to present and discuss research findings concerning the associations between sensory impairment and mental health. Focus will be on two different explanations: First, common genetic or neurological components may cause both sensory impairment and mental health problems. Second that sensory impairment affects communicative abilities, social interaction, and limits input from the surrounding environment, all of which may increase the individual's level of stress in everyday life. Research in correlation between sensory impairment and mental health issues is important both in order to better understand the impact of sensory impairment on human functioning and to gain more knowledge about mental health and sensation in general. The chapter starts with a review of existing research regarding the prevalence of mental health problems in persons with visual impairment, hearing impairment, and dual sensory loss, respectively. Mental health issues of special interest will be elaborated upon according to type of sensory impairment, for example cases of depression among elderly people with acquired deaf-blindness and cases of autism among children with congenital blindness. A major topic will be discussions of how communication and language difficulties following sensory impairment are associated with mental health problems. For children, in particular, sensory impairment may result in language delays that may have serious consequences for their development. Finally, clinical issues will be discussed, for example challenges regarding assessment, differential diagnostics, and recommended treatment procedures. In conclusion, sensory impairment, in most cases, is not a direct cause to mental health problems but is a contributing factor to an increased vulnerability towards developing mental health disorders. Communication and language development are found to be one of the most important components in prevention and treatment of mental health problems among individuals with sensory impairment.

Chapter 3 – *Background:* An epidemiological transition hypothesis has been theoretically developed and substantiated using one measure of socio-economic status (gross national domestic product [GDP]) to simultaneously explain wide cross-national variations in elderly suicide rates, trends over time for elderly suicide rates and age-associated trends in suicides rates. A curvilinear (inverted U-shaped curve) relationship between elderly suicide rates and GDP fitting the quadratic equation $Y = A + BX - CX^2$ (where Y is the suicide rate, X is the GDP and A,B, and C are constants) has been observed in a large cross-national study. *Methods:* The predicted curvilinear relationship between elderly suicide rates and the Gini coefficient, another measure of socio-economic status (income inequality), fitting the above quadratic equation was examined with curve estimation regression model using data from the World Health Organisation. *Results:* The relationship between suicide rates in both sexes in the age-bands 65-74 and 75+ years and the Gini coefficient was curvilinear and fitted the above quadratic equation, and was statistically significant (at least $P<0.05$) in all four groups. *Conclusions:* Caution should be exercised in accepting this model of the epidemiological transition hypothesis for elderly suicide rates because it was generated from cross-sectional data using an ecological design. However, the previously observed relationship was replicated by using a different measure of socio-economic status. Ideally, this model requires rigorous testing by following selected low socio-economic status countries, over time, as they develop socio-economically.

Chapter 4 – Pellagra is a systemic disease resulting from decreased cellular niacin and clinically presenting with the diagnostic triad of dermatitis, diarrhoea and dementia ('three Ds'). Although infrequently described in the pellagra literature, a number of neuropsychiatric symptoms other than dementia may present at any stage of the disease and affect a large proportion of patients. These include anxiety, depression and mania, as well as hallucinations, disturbances of thought and delusional beliefs. A number of personality changes have also been reported, resulting in social isolation, violence and aggression. Finally, *ante litteram* Parkinsonian features have been identified since the earliest description of pellagra. In addition to the neuropsychiatric symptoms that may result from the disease, it should also be noted that certain psychiatric conditions, such as anorexia nervosa and alcohol dependence, may be the underlying reason for the dietary deficiency. Cases of pellagra are not rare in developing countries and may be on the increase in the developed world. It is important to consider the full neuropsychiatric spectrum of pellagra, particularly since a number of patients may present with a clinical picture which does not exactly match the 'classical' diagnostic triad (e.g. *pellagra sine pellagra*).

In: Mental Health and Psychiatry ISBN: 978-1-62417-589-3
Editors: A.S. Wilson and M.S. Schneider

Chapter 1

COGNITIVE AND EMOTIONAL PROCESSES IN APPROACHING PERSONALITY DISORDERS

Miguel A. Pérez-Nieto, Francisco López-Muñoz [*] ***and Marta M. Redondo***

Department of Psychology, Faculty of Health Sciences, Camilo José Cela University, Madrid, Spain

ABSTRACT

This chapter review the key role played by basic psychological processes in the current conceptualization of personality disorders, the most outstanding models, and the cognitive-behavioral therapies. Currently, there is an increasing tendency towards more dimensional approaches at the expense of more categorical ones. Basic psychological processes are more relevant for dimensional approaches. In this regard, a number of models will be described: the 7 factor model, the Big Five model, the biosocial model, and the cognitive models. Likewise, the basics of both cognitive-behavioral approaches to personality disorders will be outlined. Finally, the role of perception, attention, memory, learning, impulsiveness, emotion, and the way cognitive-behavioral therapies cope with them will also be reviewed. All these processes should be given due relevance.

---

[*] Corresponding author: F. López-Muñoz, MD, PhD. E-mail: flopez@ucjc.edu.

Keywords: Personality disorders, Cognitive processes, Impulsiveness, Emotion, Cognitive-behavioural therapy

According to the DSM-IV-TR, personality disorders are defined as stable and inflexible patterns of behaviour and inner experience (cognitive and affective processes) that deviate significantly from the cultural expected, which extend from adolescence or beginning of adulthood and are a source of social maladjustment or discomfort (APA, 2000). It is precisely the permanence of the maladjusted cognitive and affective processes, which separates there disorders from the ones of clinic character and thus forces the diagnostic classification to generate a parallel axis.

This discrimination appeared in the DSM-III (APA, 1980) and was and is still understood as an advance in diagnostic classification, however, after more than 20 years, this conceptualisation of personality disorders has not reached to be fully satisfying and valid for all the scientific community, of whom still arise critiques about communality, the overlap and a certain arbitrariness in the domains that cluster the different disorders (see Livesley, 2003; Millon, 2002; Tyrer et al., 2007; Widiger and Samuel, 2005).

This critiques, added to the presence of works, which demonstrate the evidence about the dimensionality of personality disorders (Trull and Durrett, 2005), or the theoretic implications of the comorbidity between the axis (Krueger, 2005) has favoured new proposals, which challenge a more simple vision about the stability of personality disorders (Clark, 2005; Shea and Yen, 2003; Tyrer et al., 2007). Clark (2007) aims a new conceptualisation of the personality disorders (PD) in which the concept of stability would be diminished, in the way that personality disorders would reflect similar combinations of personality patterns (O`Connor, 2002, 2005) as such they would represent a rather moderate stability, but would differ in intensity, inadaptability and behavioural consequences.

In summary, personality disorders would be defined as acute symptoms linked to maladaptive patterns (e.g. interpersonal avoidance) and/or defensive or compensatory behaviours, which present themselves in internal and/or external coping processes (Skodol et al., 2005). The richness of dimensional approaches in personality disorders and the derived benefits of such approaches seem to have influenced, although just to some extent, the reformulation of personality disorders that are seen in the drafts of the future DSM-V. In the new diagnostic version of personality disorders will be included, besides specific references to the capacity of adaptation of the individual, a series of six patterns and domains clearly dimensional (Esbec and Echeburúa, 2011). In our opinion, this approach favours an approximation rather attending to the performance of basic psychological processes of personality disorders, which is, attending especially to the performance of processes involved in cognitive, affective and behavioural areas.

Evidence about the existence of personality dimension shave helped a lot in this direction and as Widiger and Mullins-Sweatt (2007) pointed out, that a good part of maladaptive personality patterns, which are included in the diagnostic criteria of personality disorders, were observed in persons, which never have obtained such a diagnostic. This, in turn, favours considering, that parts of the symptoms of PD could be variants of personality patterns included in general theoretical models about personality (Saulsman and Page, 2004; Widiger and Costa, 2002).

This rather dimensional posture is not necessarily opposed, if attending to proposals like the one from Millon and Escovar (1996) which based in the concept of "prototype", identifies the individual, which possesses all the characteristics of one category, but assuming, that this would be the extreme of a vector, which would help to define diagnostically those cases with high comorbidity in between the different diagnostic categories which currently exist. Lynam and Widiger (2001) developed a "prototype" method of PD diagnostics according to the Big five model, finding some studies with a good fit of the expert system for identifying prototypes and the current Big Five model (Miller, Reynolds and Pilkonis, 2004). In any case, an approximation towards personality disorders, which gives relevance to the aggravation of some personality dimensions, has the consequence, in our opinion, that the affective, cognitive and behavioural processes, which allow identifying this aggravation, will be the truly objective of the intervention.

Thereby, as some investigations in the case of borderline personality disorder for example demonstrate (Morey and Zanarini, 2000; Trull et al., 2003), that the symptoms could be basically seen as extreme versions of anger, anxiety, depression, impulsiveness and/or vulnerability, all of them belonging, in the scope of emotions, to negative affect or negative emotionality and in the scope of personality, to neuroticism.

Ultimately, the identification of both, cognitive and affective processes, as well as emotional and motivational ones, common to diverse explanatory models of personality disorders, as well as their impact in different specific therapies for personality disorders, will be the objective of the current paper. With this, it is intended to stimulate the identification of therapeutic objectives in different interventions, adapting those to the processes, which will become symptoms. Anyhow, there must be taken into account that the cognitive, affective and behavioural processes, which are identified as symptoms can be generators and maintainers of the disorder itself, like it occurs in purely clinic disorders or in the development of personality starting from non-linear dynamic models (Lewis, 2000).

PERSONALITY MODELS

In the explanation about the structure and the development of the personality, both approaches are combined, on the one hand, approximations of a rather biological character, whose factors are named temperamental, and on the other hand rather environmental approximations, whose factors are named characterological (Caballo, 2004). The influence of biological variables in the behavioural regulation is attached to the development of psychology as a science and authors like Paulov already hypothesized about mechanism of alternation and the balance between "basic processes of stimulation and inhibition" (Olivencia and Cangas, 2002).

Although there is a big body of models existing, which are important and could be highlighted in the explanation of personality, its structure and the basic processes, like learning, affect and emotion, etc. (e.g. Eysenck, 1991; Gray, 1981; Livesley and Jackson, 1999; Watson and Tellegen, 1985), we will just analyse some of the them, which we have considered the most influential in the clinical approach. Nowadays, one of the most relevant theoretical models, which gives special importance to temperamental variables, is the seven factors model of Cloninger (1998, 2000).

The model suggests four temperamental dimensions, which reflect innate dispositions of stimulus response, which are persistent over time and on the other hand the model also suggests three characterological dimensions, which reflect individual differences acquired in non-linear interactions within character disposition and vital experiences (Svrakic et al., 2002).

The temperamental dimensions suggested in the model of Cloninger are: "novelty seeking", which refers to behavioural activation; "harm avoidance", which refers to behavioural inhibition; "reward dependence", which refers to the processes of extinction and habituation of learned behavioural responses; and lastly, a fourth dimension, which initially belonged to "reward dependence", which is called "persistence".

For the first three dimensions Cloninger stated the hypothesis, that each one of the first three dimensions of temperament would be associated respectively to a determinate neurotransmitter monoamine, which would be dopamine for "novelty seeking", serotonin for "harm avoidance" and noradrenalin for "reward dependence".

According to the three character dimensions, they would be: "cooperativeness" (empathy facing hostility); "self-transcendence" (authenticity and imagination about control); and "self-directedness" which refers to the capacity maintaining a behaviour following an objective while facing insecurity, which is, the capacity to auto-regulate behaviour.

In line with the dimensions proposed by Cloninger, a personality disorder emerges through acquiring low levels of "cooperativeness", "self-transcendence" and specially "self-directedness", linking the type of personality disorder to each of the four temperament types. A revision and detailed description of the general model and particularly the biological foundation, can be read in a recent published chapter by the author of the model (Cloninger, 2007).

In this perspective, which includes rather temperamental dimensions, can be located as well the models of normal personality, like the "big five" model (Costa and McCrae, 1985), which derives from a factorial development, beginning with a lexical analysis, presenting a high diffusion and utilization as well in the evaluation and diagnostics of personality disorders, although presenting some limitations in those aspects (Bagby, Costa, Widiger, Ryder and Marshall, 2005; Furnam and Crump, 2005). The five dimensions that proposes the model are: "neuroticism", "extraversion", "openness", "agreeableness" and "conscientiousness" (compromise with the objective), have shown certain degree of association with some of the dimensions of the model from Cloninger (see Farabaugh et al., 2005). The character, by defining itself as learned dimensions linked to psychosocial factors, tends to form itself in a continuous way, but especially in the most basic processes of socialisation.

Among the models focused in character dimensions, stand out the ones focusing on the concept of "scheme". Schemes are structured, criss-crossed systems, which are responsible for the processing of a perceived stimulus and it is associated behavioural response (Beck et al., 1995). A very descriptive definition of Segal (1998) would be „organized elements of past experiences and reactions, which form a fairly compact body and persistent knowledge which is able to direct post- perceptions and – evaluations."

These schemes can influence the evaluation process and also skew them. The identification of characteristic schemes for each type of personality disorder has been a fundamental element in the cognitive approach of personality disorders. Although always with a rather therapeutic than explanatory intention, being nowadays the "schemes therapy" of Young (1999), with not just applying a cognitive vision, had identified more relevant and better schemes in personality disorders.

Facing the diversity of the theoretic models derived from the distinct perspectives, which tackle the personality and its disorders, different authors have searched for integrated models (see Escovar, 1997; Paris, 1996). The approach which nowadays gained major degree of integration and diffusion is the "evolutionary model" from Millon (1990), in which, besides including cognitive, behavioural and biological aspects, takes as well account on some interpersonal (see Kiesler, 1982; Benjamin, 1996) and psychodynamic perspectives (see Abraham, 1927; Fenichel, 1945; Kermberg, 1996). This model has it's beginning in a previous version, the model of the "bio-social learning theory" (Millon, 1985), in which Millon gave similar effects to the biological and psychosocial variables towards personality, combining the theoretical approach "nature of reinforcement" (positive, negative or none) and the "origin of reinforcement" (me, others, ambivalent, aligned) with the "instrumental behaviour" (active or passive).

Based on these variables, a taxonomy of biosocial learning, which combines the active-passive dimension with four other styles, is established: independent, dependent, ambivalent and detached. The current model of Millon extracts of the psychodynamic, cognitive, interpersonal and biologic perspectives, eight areas of manifestation of personality: defence mechanism, object representations, self-image, cognitive style, interpersonal behaviour and mood/temperament. In a previous level to this expression of personality are located the polarities which structure them, the four dimensions or "spheres" are: "pleasure-pain", "passivity or accommodation to the environment vs. activity or modification of the environment", "myself- others" and "high vs. low abstraction".

COGNITIVE BEHAVIOURAL TREATMENT

As Pretzer and Beck (2004) point it out, the cognitive-behavioural treatment of personality disorders is especially relevant, among others, due to the reason, that those disorders are every time more defined in cognitive and behavioural terms, and a large part of cognitive-behavioural treatments are applied to patients with a 50% comorbidity with alterations of the personality

(Turkat and Maisto, 1985), more present, for instance, in patients with chronic depression (Prieto, Vera, Pérez and Ramírez, 2007).

The effectiveness of cognitive-behavioural interventions for personality disorders varies greatly along the different disorders, being the most effective in the Borderline Personality Disorder, Avoidant Personality Disorder and Dependent Personality Disorder and less effective in the Schizoid, Antisocial and Narcissistic Personality disorders (Caballo, 2001).

In accordance with the revision of Quiroga and Errasti (2001), the classical behavioural therapy and the dialectical behavioural therapy – DBT from Linehan (1993a) are the only ones with sufficient empirical proof to be likely efficient in treating borderline personality disorder.

Thus, as being empirically proven, in the next section the principles and phases of DBT will be discussed, and, as well the Scheme Therapy (Young, 1999; Young, Klosk and Weishaar, 2003) for being under extensive development. There will be no emphasis about classical behavioural therapy, as it is assumed to be known.

Dialectical Behavioural Therapy – DBT

The DBT developed itself as a treatment for the Borderline Personality Disorder – BPT- with suicidal and self-damaging tendency, starting off as an explanatory model for these disorders from the Biosocial Theory of Millon. In this context the BPT is seen as a disorder in which the capacity of auto-regulation of emotions, behaviour, cognition and interpersonal relations is altered. This alteration in the regulation, in accordance with the Biosocial Model, is due to innate emotional vulnerability and a disabling childhood environment (Linehan, 1993a).

The DBT is fundamentally based in learning principles, in the classic conditioning, as well as in the operant conditioning, leaving behind cognition on a second level and considering it as another behavior (Stanley and Brodsky, 2007). To these principles Linehan adds the “mindfulness” concept and a dialectic approach. With the “mindfulness” orientation it is intended to take into account that current maladaptive behaviours (e.g. autolysis) as the best ones available till the moment, when they will be changed without necessity to change.

This rather eastern philosophy – zen (Robins, 2002), favours a more dialectic approach in the cognitive restructuration, which would be rather oriented towards adding new strategies, than changing already existing ones, which tackles as well the polarized thinking, which is common in BPD. In fact, the dialectic approach defines itself, by trying to link opposites, which are dichotomies, and thus being the basis for three assumptions for therapy: the patients collaborate the best way possible; the patients cannot have caused all their problems and have tried to solve them; and the patients cannot fail, just the treatment can. With this assumption, the DBT is divided in four different phases (Linehan, 1993b), which in turn includes different modules. A general structure would be the following:

- Phase I: "Mindfulness".
  - Focus in the moment.
  - Consciousness without critiques.
- Phase II: Tolerance to the "pain":
  - Strategy to survive a crisis
  - Radical acceptation of the reality
- Phase III: Emotional regulation
  - Observe and identify emotional states
  - Validate and accept own emotions
  - Reduce vulnerability towards negative emotions
  - Increase the experience of positive emotions
- Phase IV: Personal effectiveness
  - Assertiveness training
  - Cognitive Reconstruction
  - Balance between objectives and maintenance of relationships and self-esteem

It is interesting to emphasise the therapeutic objectives, which were set in the first phase, for hierarchical condition, which is the first place force to reduce parasuicidal behaviour, and in second place, reduce behaviours, which interfere with therapy, and in third place, reduce behaviours, which interfere with quality of life (Stanley and Brodsky, 2007). These objectives have to be kept in mind, while removing critiques and focusing in the current moment.

According to the objective of the present work, it seems interesting to stress the objective processes of phase three of emotional regulation. In this phase, the emotional response and its vulnerability are regulated by focusing on biological, cognitive, and behavioural processes. In the biological processes, specific skills, like the "PLEASE" skill, which focuses in the optimization of the physical area, food, drug consumption, sleeping patterns and physical exercise, are included. For the cognitive processes implicated in the emotional response, performance via attentional processes and its evaluation is included, as well as self-knowledge and meta-cognition. An extensive and recently published revision about emotional auto-regulation and its foundations in the DBT can be found in Linehan, Bohus and Lynch (2007).

In the beginning the DBT was examined in a clinical controlled study with a randomly selected sample (Linehan et al., 1991; Linehan, Heard and Armstrong, 1993; Linehan et al., 1994; Shearin and Linehan, 1994). The results showed, after treatment of one year compared to regular treatment, clinical positive and significant effects in three relevant areas: suicidal behaviour and automutilation; permanence in the treatment and quantity of hospital treatments.

Scheme Therapy (ST)

The Scheme Therapy and the DBT have quite a lot in common, even if it does not seem on first sight, but the both coincide in fundamental aspects like the balance between acceptance and confrontation strategies (Klosko and Young, 2004).

The therapy integrates distinct cognitive-behavioural techniques in one methodological body, besides including more recent techniques from other similar approaches, starting with a causal analysis of the patient's beliefs and cognitive distortions (Valenzuela and Caballo, 2001).

The Scheme Therapy raised as an answer to the limitations of the classic cognitive therapy for personality disorders (Beck and Freeman, 1990) and is based in the cognitive therapy of Beck for depression (Beck, Rush, Shaw and Emery, 1979). The reformulated model of Beck for personality understands it as specific patterns of social, motivational, cognitive and emotional processes, which are determinate by its idiosyncratic structure and can be defined as a scheme and be represented by nuclear beliefs (Alford and Beck, 1997).

The Schemes Therapy treats those topics and central beliefs of the patient with personality disorder, by labelling them as "early maladaptive schemes", which are the starting point in therapy. According to Young and Klosko (2007), an early maladaptive scheme is understood as "a scheme compound of memories, emotions, cognitions and body sensations in relation with one self, and the relationships from one with other persons, which developed during childhood or puberty, intensified during the life of an individual and dysfunctional in a significant degree".

This schemes are supposed to have their origin in an interaction of not satisfied central emotional needs in the childhood and temperamental characteristics, which are biological and innate, as a child, five emotional needs are seen as central: secure affect with other persons, autonomy, competence and sense of identity, the freedom to express needs and valid emotions, spontaneity and play, realistic boarders and self-control. The early maladaptive schemes, which will be discussed, are as well five, even if with different domains associated, it would lead to a total of 18 specific identified schemes in this therapy. The basic five are termed after the following sections 1) early disconnection and rejection; 2) autonomy and performance disorder; 3) altered boundaries; 4) being guided by others; and 5) hypervigilance and inhibition. A detailed description of the schemes in Spanish can be found in Young and Klosko (2007). It is important to mention, that the therapy distinguish between maladaptive schemes and the coping strategy, which is used to confront such a scheme. Thereby, coping strategies can be varied for oneself and as well along the time, beginning to confront the scheme with one type of behaviour and varying afterwards to others. Ultimately, scheme therapy points out three basic styles of maladaptive coping of the schemes, which by themselves are maladaptive: the surrender to the scheme, the avoidance of the scheme and the activation of the scheme as an overcompensation of the scheme.

The combination of one scheme and one coping style in a certain moment is what the therapy calls "mode". Examples of modes or specific coping responses in relation with maladaptive schemes can be found in Young and Klosko (2007). In the schemes therapy the psychologist seeks with empathy, to change those modes generating coping styles for its corresponding schemes, which will be adaptive and does not include surrender, avoidance and overcompensation.

The schemes therapy therefore structures beliefs and coping styles, which are based in emotions, auto-cognitions and maladaptive learning. Nowadays the schemes therapy has a wide diffusion and has received great reliability and internal consistence for schemes identified of the same (see Schmidt et al., 1995), and even though data about its efficiency is missing, some studies (Young and Klosko, 2007) show a higher efficiency in the treatment of Borderline Personality Disorder. Lastly, the schemes therapy can be considered as an evolution and development of the cognitive therapy for personality disorders.

Basic Processes in Personality Disorders, Models and Cognitive-behavioural Therapies

It can be especially relevant, to identify the basic components of cognitive, learning, motivational and emotional processes in personality disorders, even more, if they role they are having in theoretical models and cognitive-behavioural therapy is analysed. To determine such a processes allows to define central elements in therapeutic process and assigning them an own entity in therapy. Hence, the literature about certain processes will be revised: attention and perception, learning, memory, emotion and motivation.

Perception

Till now basic processes like attention and perception have not received much prominence in the research of PD, neither in explanatory models, nor in revised therapeutic approaches.

Just a view studies have investigated perceptual processes, although some investigations, for instance Bohus et al. (2000), demonstrate significant variations in the threshold of pain perception in borderline disorder patients, indicating that the threshold increases in stress situations till it reaches an important level of analgesic function in self-damaging behaviour, and decreasing significantly in the absence of such stressors (Schmahl, Meinzer, Zeuch, 2010; Reitz, Krause-Utz, Pogatzki-Zahn, Ebner-Priemer, Bohus, and Schmahl; 2012).

In personality disorders, the patients perception of time seems altered as well, which results in an increased subjective sensation of velocity (Berlin and Rolls, 2004). In patients with schizotypal personality disorder was found a deficit in the visual perception and the processing of such information in comparison with schizophrenic patients (Farmer, O`Donnell, Niznikiewicz, Voglmaier, McCarley and Shenton, 2000).

As well the perception of interpersonal behaviors was object of investigation, but, for example in the perception and identification of aggression, which is understood as a violent reaction, no differences in PD were detected (Muro, Tomás, Moreno and Rubio, 2002).

Attention

There have been found difficulties in the sensorial integration for patients with schizotypal personality disorder (Cadenhead, Light, Geyer and Braff, 2000), but as well in borderline patients, in whose the attentional alterations have been linked in a greater extend to personality alterations, identifying some works which highlighted the connection between the history of attention deficit disorder and the presence of a borderline personality disorder (see Flory et al., 2007; Fossati, Novella, Donati, Donini and Maffei, 2002), a disorder in which attentional patterns play an highly important role (Wingenfeld, Mensebach, Rullkoetter et al. 2009).

To be more precisely, authors like Sieswerda and its team have pointed out the relevance that attention can play in personality disorders in general, although especially in borderline personality disorders and the therapeutic process (Arntz, Apples and Sieswerda, 2000; Sieswerda, Arntz, Mertens and Vertoment, 2007). This research team has investigated the selective attention with the emotional stroop paradigm, finding higher levels of hypervigilance and attentional biases towards threatening stimuli in patients with borderline personality, with hypervigilance reducing significantly in those borderline patients who obtain therapeutic success (Sieswerda, Arntz and Kindt, 2007). Likewise, attention appears explicitly emphasised as a part of the therapeutic process in phase III of DBT, in which the attentional display is stimulated (Linehan, Bohus and Lynch, 2007).

Learning and Memory

The learning processes in classic conditioning and operant conditioning are clearly integrated in the most relevant explanatory model of PD, as well in the most temperamental or biological one from Cloninger, and of course, in the one with bigger emphasis on socialisation, from Milon.

Its interesting to highlight, that in the seven factors model of Cloninger, the temperament is linked to an associative/procedural learning and the learning character is seen as reflexive and includes the memory as well (Heim and Westen, 2007). So, in the temperament, one of its dimensions is the "dependence on reward", which is the reinforcement, and other, which is "avoidance of harm", clearly linked to the concept of negative reinforcement. Obviously, the biosocial learning model from Millon gives special protagonism to the reinforcement, in referring to its nature, itself, and the instrumental behaviour, which form the three initial polarities.

As well in the therapeutic approach, revising the learning and memory processes becomes important, being especially relevant the principles of classic and operant conditioning in the DBT of Linehan and assuming fundamental the well-functioning of the memory and its different structures in the schemes therapy of Young. To be more specific, the classic conditioning is used in the identification of possible associative deficits in psychopathy and antisocial personality, finding limitations especially in those subjects in anticipating aversive events (Birbaumer et al., 2005; Flor, Birbaumer, Hermann, Ziegler and Patrick, 2002).

In this population, besides the association difficulties, memory problems in the recuperation of emotional damaging information is assumed, focusing research in the activity of the prefrontal-limbic- cortex circuit (Dolan and Fullam, 2005).

The operative memory is subject of studies especially in the context of schizotypal personality disorders, where evidence shows a worse performance in the processing of visual and auditive information, with clear deficits in the episodic memory (Farmer et al., 2000; McClure, Romero, Bowie, Reichenberg, Harvey and Siever, 2007; Mitropoulou, Harvey, Zegarelli, New, Silverman and Siever, 2005). In the borderline personality disorder, the functioning of the operative memory was investigated as well, finding, again, a worse performance of the operative memory in the velocity to process sensory information (Stevens, Burkhardt, Hautzinger, Schwarz and Unckel, 2004).

In the same disorder (BPD) the autobiographical memory was subject of research, with some studies indicating a certain deficit in the activation of areas involved in the autobiographic memory, which suggests a self-referring tendency in the processing of the information (Schnell, Dietrich, Schnitker, Daumann and Herpertz, 2007).

However, it is important to point out, that other work does not indicate differences between control groups and borderline patients in the use of self-referring memory in processing items with emotional content (Minzenberg, Fisher-Irving, Poole and Vinogradov, 2006). Traumatic contents are well remembered by borderline patients (Kremers et al., 2007), although the presence of depressive symptoms favours the occurrence of errors in the episodic memory (Kremers, Spinhoven and Van der Does, 2004).

Emotion and Impulsiveness

The emotional processes are highly relevant in the PD, as being the affective domain one out of four diagnostic areas in which any diagnostic in PD is based.

Likewise, the emotional responses are not just describing and categorizing the different personality disorders, but also they are fundamental elements in the therapeutic process, especially in the DBT, in which a whole treatment phase is assigned to the emotional regulation and response, and as such being the core objective for some authors (García Palacios, 2006).

The scheme therapy acts similar, thus, unresolved emotional needs are seen at the base of an issue, coping strategies, which have to be cultivated, try to regulate the emotional response.

Still, in the revised explanatory models, there is not explicitly relevance given to the emotional processes, like for example, the auto-regulation of emotional responses, despite the obvious value of such processes in the therapeutic setting and the relevance of emotional responses in the description, categorization and diagnostics of PD and in the dimensional conceptualization of them.

In an implicit way, however, the emotional processes have presence in both models, in the model of Millon, and the model of Coninger, as both include a dimension which is called "sensation seeking", which for Millon represents a polarity of the affective nature "pleasure-pain", and for Cloninger it contains motivational variables, like exploration, as well as impulsiveness.

Impulsiveness is probably one of the emotional/motivational elements, which transversely got most relevance in the cognitive-behavioural approach in PD, being a fundamental variable in the borderline personality. The connection between emotional responses and impulsiveness is very strong in PD. Impulsiveness is a variable, which because of interfering in the control of emotional and behavioural regulation processes, plays an important role in the development of various psychological alterations, among them: addiction, bipolar disorder, impulse control disorder and especially, disorders of the cluster B of PD. The conceptual delimitation of impulsiveness is not easy, although in its definition, delimitation and comprehension are usually included concepts as well as conceptual disinhibition and aggression, the role of habituation processes and extinction towards reinforcement and punishment, as well as underlying biological foundations. Revisions about the topic can be found in García Marco (2004) and Arranz, García Blanco and Ros Montalbán (2004).

Nonetheless, a clear linkage between impulsiveness and behavioural disinhibition can be assumed, as a linkage with greater dependence on more intense and immediate reinforcement, which would give to the emotion a greater importance as a "reason" for subsequent behaviour (Pérez Nieto, Redondo, Sánchez Burón and Fernández, 2007). The borderline personality has been the field in which most studies about emotional deregulation and impulsiveness have been applied. According to the emotional deregulation, findings have contributed to the existence of a neural substrate, specifically, the frontal-limbic system which is associated to the emotional and behavioural decontrol (Silbersweig et al., 2007; Williams, Sidis, Gordon and Meares, 2006), although in the context of rather biological approximations, and as well from the "Polyvagal Theory" (Porges, 1995), the emotional deregulation is explained (Austin, Riniolo and Porges, 2007).

However, when an exam of emotional deregulation in borderline patients is done, variables like the tolerance towards stress can change clearly the scope of the deregulation, the more, the higher the stress (Gratz, Rosenthal, Tull, Legues and Gunderson, 2006). Impulsiveness is a characteristic variable in personality disorders of group B, but as well in group A and C of PD can be found clinical relevant impulsive responses, in fact, the impulse control disorder and PD shared the same categorization till the DSV-III (Szerman, 2004), leading in the 1980ies to propose a "multi-impulsive personality disorder" (Lacey and Evans, 1986). Yet, impulsiveness represents a fundamental variable in the group B disorders, as well by presenting itself as a variable, which could explain the high degree of co-variation in the disorders representing this group (Fossati, Barratt, Borrón, Villa, Grazioli and Maffei, 2007).

Actually, impulsiveness is one of the elements, which seems to explain as well the association between the disorders of group B and substance abuse (Casillas and Clark, 2002), presenting themselves, impulsiveness and substance abuse, as one dimension with the explanatory capacity for PD (Besteiro, Lemos, Muñiz, García and Álvarez, 2007). Still, even though the link between disorders of group B and substance abuse mediating impulsiveness is assumed, the multi-dimensional nature of impulsiveness forces to deepen in its nuances and some works point out the important role of negative emotionality in this variable and context, enhancing its consequences (Bornovalova, Legues, Daughters, Rosenthal and Lynch, 2005).

Similarly, the relationship between disorders of group B (e.g. the anti-social or the borderline personality) and violence, present themselves clearly linked to the role of impulsiveness (see Komarovskaya, López and Warren,

2007; Retz, Retz-Junginger, Supprian, Thome and Rosler, 2004), being in a lot of cases the affective instability and a certain emotional responses, which favour the disinhibition of such behaviours.

Emotional labiality and impulsiveness, both common in the borderline and bipolar disorders (Henry, Mitropoulou, New, Koenigsberg, Silverman and Siever, 2001) display the importance of regulation of certain emotional responses. Emotional responses, which mostly appear in PD are anger, fear/anxiety and sadness. Nevertheless, speaking of anxiety and depression in this context implies usually exploring the clinical picture, which not just includes one emotional response, but various (like anger and sadness in an depressive episode), and a trajectory and associated behaviours, which would surpass the objective of this paper, and are therefore not included in this revision.

According to basic emotional responses, there have been taken place attempts to integrate anger and fear to the wide affective and behavioural spectrum of PD (Lara, Pinto, Akiskal and Akiskal, 2006), and as well, linking the theory of discrete emotions to the symptoms of borderline personality disorder, giving special emphasis to anger and fear (Magai and Hunziker, 1998). However, it must be said, even if the diagnostic of any PD makes reference to some specific emotional response, the chance that the same will be objective of study to structure the disorder, is low, being auto-regulation processes, the ones which have taken account of this important role.

Cognitive Contents, Evaluation and Coping

Enough evidence exists, especially regarding to cluster C, about the importance of the interpretation bias (Arntz, Weertman and Salet, 2011). Cognitive contents and coping processes enjoy protagonism in explanatory models and in revised cognitive-behavioural therapies.

In the seven-factors model of Cloninger "self-directedness" and "self-transcendence" are included as dimensions, which form the realm of character. Millon includes as well the abstraction process as another "sphere" in his personality styles, implicitly making reference to the coping processes with its active-passive dimension.

In this cognitive processes occurs as well agreement on a therapeutic level, in the way that, especially in the schemes therapy, which clearly assumes the relevance of cognitive content, reaches to "define them" according to disorders which start from prototypical beliefs for schemes. This therapy includes as well specific reference to coping, pointing out three specific styles to develop a PD. In this therapy, evaluation processes would be applied as well for re-construction. In the DBT, evaluation processes are the ones, which are explicitly marked as part of the therapeutic process in phase III, favouring the situational re-evaluation (Linehan, Bohus and Lynch, 2007), besides giving special importance to the emotional regulation as a emotional coping process, and by beginning treatment with acceptance as a clear coping strategy.

DISCUSSION

Thus, the cognitive processes of evaluation, coping, beliefs and cognitive contents are those in which the cognitive-behavioural approach of PD is based on to a bigger extent, although always giving special importance to the contents, being easy to find research which identifies beliefs associated to the disorders (see Arntz, Dreessen, Schouten and Weertman, 2004; Jones, Burell-Hodgson and Tate, 2007).

Nonetheless, in prior works the role of such cognitive processes and others like attention, memory or the thinking process in PD in general (Pérez Nieto, González Ordi and Redondo, 2007) or, in particular, the borderline personality (Baer, Peters, Eishenlhor-Moul, Geiger and Seuer, 2012), have been revised. Though, the most relevant models and therapies in the cognitive-behavioural context reveal the importance of the formation of these beliefs, styles, ways, etc., which could be the top of the iceberg, giving however, less attention to processes involved in its formation and maintenance. Thereby, variables which are linked to meta-cognitive processing are included, for example the "self-directedness·of Cloninger or the identification schemes in oneself, but there is no theoretic body about those processes applied to disorders, although it already exists for anxiety disorders (see Wells, 2000). Meta-cognitive beliefs can have an effect in the use of certain strategies of cognitive and impulsiveness control (Pérez-Nieto, Redondo and Martin, 2005; Pérez-Nieto et al., 2007), aspects, which in turn are fundamental in the emotional regulation, where there seems to exist a greater deepening.

The emotional regulation presents itself as highly relevant in the therapeutic setting, as much as in schemes therapy, as especially in DBT, where the emotional regulation occupies a wide part of the therapy and from where also attentional, valorational, activational, etc. processes implied in the appearance of the emotional response, are departing (Linehan, Bohus and Lynch, 2007).

Once the limitations of categorical models compared to dimensional models of PD are taken into account, arises an approach of the same from a non-linear dynamic models perspective, which assumes continuous processes over the time (see Bornas and García de la Banda, 2001); and that the most promising therapies focus in emotional, motivational and behavioural processes to reach therapeutic success, it can be now the moment in which the dimensional approach bases itself in the most basic processes. The complexity of PD and the rare efficiency of therapies for those can be seen as fighting against the identification of the most relevant processes and the development of specific strategies for its regulation.

REFERENCES

Abraham, K. (1927). The influence of oral erotism on character formation. In C.A.D. Bryan and A. Strachey (Eds.), *Selected papers on psychoanalysis*. London: Hogarth.

Alford, B.A. and Beck, A.T. (1997).*The integrative power of cognitive therapy*. New York: Guilford Press.

American Psychiatric Association (1980).*Diagnostic and Statistical Manual of Mental Disorders-Third Edition. (DSM-III)*. Washington, DC: APA.

American Psychiatric Association (2000).*Diagnostic and Statistical Manual of Mental Disorders-Fourth Edition.Text revission (DSM-IV-TR)*. Washington, DC: APA

Arntz, A., Appels, C., Sieswerda, S. (2000). Hypervigilance in borderline disorder: A test with the emotional Stroop paradigm. *Journal of Personality Disorders*, 14, 363-377.

Arntz, A., Weertman, A., and Salet, A. (2011) Interpretation bias in Cluster-C and borderline personality disorders. *Behaviour Research and Therapy*, 49, 472–481.

Arranz Estévez, F.J., García Blanco, S. and Ros Montalbán, S. (2004). Modelos experimentales de investigación de la impulsividad. In S. Ros Montalbán, M.D. Peris Díaz and R. Gracia Marco (Eds.), *Impulsividad* (pp. 23-39). Barcelona: Ars Medica.

Austin, M.A., Riniolo, T.C., and Porges, S.W. (2007). Borderline personalitydisorder and emotion regulation: Insights from the Polyvagal Theory. *Brain and Cognition,* 65, 69-76.

Baer, R.A., Peters, J.R., Eisenlohr-Moul, T.A., Geiger, P.J., and Sauer, S.E. (2012). Emotion-related cognitive processes in borderline personality disorder: a review of the empirical literature. *Clinical Psychology Review,* 32, 359-369.

Bagby, R.M., Costa, P.T., Widiger, T.A., Ryder, A.G., and Marshall, M. (2005). DSM-IV personality disorders and the five-factor model of personality: a multi-method examination of domain and facet-level predictions. *European Journal of Personality,* 19, 307-324.

Beck, A.T. (1976). *Cognitive therapy and the emotional disorders.* London: Penguin Books.

Beck, A.T. and Freeman, A. (1990). *Cognitive therapy of the personality disorders.* New York: Guilford Press.

Beck, A.T., Rush, a.J., Shaw, B.F. and Emery, G. (1979). *Cognitive therapy for depression.* New York: Guilfod Press.

Beck, A.T.; Freeman, A, Pretzer, J., Davis, D.D.Fleming, B., Ottaviani, R., et al. (1995). *Terapia cognitiva de los trastornos de personalidad.* Barcelona: Paidos.

Benjamin, L.S. (1996). *Interpersonal diagnosis and treatment of personality disorders.* New York: Guilford Press

Berlin, H.A. and Rolls, E.T. (2004). Time perception, impulsivity, emotionality, and personality in self-harming borderline personality disorder patients. *Journal of Personality Disorders*, 18, 358-378.

Besteiro, J., Lemos, S., Muñiz, J., García, E. and Álvarez, M. (2007).Dimensiones de los trastornos de personalidad en el MCMI-II. *Journal of Clinical and Health Psychology,* 7, 295-306.

Bohus, M., Limberger, M., Ebner, U., Glocker, F.X., Schwarz, B., Wernz, M., and Lieb, K. (2000). Pain perception during self-reported distress and calmness in patients with borderline personality disorder and self-mutilating behavior. *Psychiatric Research,* 95, 251-260.

Bornas, X. and García de la Banda, G. (2001) Trastornos de la personalidad: un enfoque desde la teoría del caos. *Psicología Conductual,* 9, 471-488.

Bornovalova,, M.A., Legues, C.W., Daughters, S.B., Rosenthal, M.Z., and Lynch, T.R. (2005). Impulsivity as a common process across borderline personality and substance use disorders. *Clinical Pscyhology Review,* 25, 790-812.

Caballo, V.E. (2001). Tratamientos cognitivo-conductuales para los trastornos de personlidad. *Psicología Conductual*, 9, 579-605.

Caballo, V.E. (2004). Conceptos actuales sobre los trastornos de personalidad. In V.E. Caballo (Ed.), *Manual de los trastornos de personalidad: descripción, evaluación y tratamiento* (pp.25-56). Madrid: Síntesis.

Cadenhead, K.S., Light, G.A., Geyer, M.A., and Braff, D.L. (2000). Sensory gating deficits assessed by the P50 event-related potential in subjects with schizotypal personality disorder. *American Journal of Psychiatry,* 157, 55-59.

Casillas, A and Clark, L.A. (2002). Dependency, impulsivity and self-harm: traits hypothesized to underlie the association between cluster B personality and substance use disorders. *Journal of Personality Disorders,* 16, 424-436.

Clark, L.A. (2005). Stability and change in personality pathology: revelations of three longitudinal studies. *Journal of Personality Disorders,* 19, 525-532.

Clark, L.A. (2007). Assessment and diagnosis of personality disorder: Perennial issues and emerging reconceptualization. *Annual Review of Psychology,* 58, 227-257.

Cloninger, C.R. (1998). The genetics and psychobiology of the seven-factor model of personality. In K.R.Silk (Eds.), *Biology of personality disorders* (pp. 63-92). Washington, DC: American Psychiatric Press.

Cloninger, C.R. (2000). A practical way to diagnosis personality disorders: a proposal. *Journal of Personality Disorders,* 14, 99-108.

Cloninger, C.R. (2007). Genética. In J.M. Oldham, A.E. Skodol and D.S. Bender (Eds.), *Tratado de los trastornos de la personalidad* (pp. 145-156). Barcelona: Elsevier Masson.

Costa, P.T. and McCrae, R.R. (1985).*The NEO Personality Inventory manual.* Odessa, FL: Psychological Assessment Resources.

Dollan, M. and Fullan, R. (2005).Memory for emotional events in violent offenders with antisocial personality disorder. *Personality and Individual Differences,* 38, 1657-1667.

Esbec, E and Echeburúa, E. (2011). New criteria for personality disorders in DSM-V. *Actas Españolas de Psiquiatría,* 39, 1-11.

Escovar, L. (1997). The Millon inventories: Socio cultural considerations. In T. Millon (Ed.), *The Millon Inventories* (pp.264-285). New York: Guilford Press.

Eysenck HJ. (1991). Dimensions of personality: the biosocial approach to personality. In J. Strelau and A. Angleitner (Eds.), *Explorations in temperament: international perspectives on theory and measurement.* London: Plenum

Farabaugh, A., Fava, M., Mischoulon, D., Sklarsky, K., Petersen, T., et al. (2005). Relationships between major depressive disorder and comorbid anxiety and personality disorders. *Comprhensive Psychiatry,* 46, 266-271.

Farmer, C.M., O'Donnell, B.F., Niznikiewicz, M.A., Voglmaier, M.M., McCarley, R.W., and Shenton, M.E. (2000). Visual perception and working memory in schizotypal personality disorder. *American Journal of Psychiatry,* 157, 781-786.

Flory, J.D., Newcorn, J.H., Miller, C., Harty, S., and Halperin, J.M. (2007). Serotonergic function in children with attention-deficit hyperactivity disorder - Relationship to later antisocial personality disorder. *British Journal of Psychiatry,* 190, 410-414.

Fossati, A., Barratt, E.S., Borroni, S., Villa, D., Grazioli, F., and Maffei, C. (2007). Impulsivity, aggressiveness and DSM-IV personality disorders. *Psychiatry Research,* 149, 157-167.

Fossati, A., Novella, L., Donati, D., Donini, M., and Maffei, C. (2002). History of childhood attention deficit/hyperactivity disorder symptoms and borderline personality disorder: A controlled study. *Comprehensive Psychiatry,* 43, 367-377.

Furnam, A. and Crump, J. (2005). Personality traits, types, and disorders: an examination of the relationship between three self-report measures. *European Journal of Personality,* 19, 167-184.

García Marco, R. (2004). Nosología de la impulsividad. In S. Ros Montalbán, M.D. Peris Díaz and R. Gracia Marco (Eds.), *Impulsividad* (pp. 15-22). Barcelona: Ars Medica.

García Palacios, A. (2006). La terapia dialéctico comportamental. *Edupykhé,* 5, 255-272.

Gratz, K.L., Rosenthal, M.Z. ,Tull, M.T., Lejuez, C.W., and Gunderson, J.G. (2006). An experimental investigation of emotion dysregulation in borderline personality disorder. *Journal of Abnormal Psychology,* 115, 850-855.

Gray JA. (1981). A critique of Eysenck's theory of personality. In H.J. Eysenck (Ed.), *A model for personality*. Berlin: Springer-Verlag,

Heim, A. and Westen, D. (2007).Teorías de la personalidad y trastornos de la personalidad. In J.M. Oldham, A.E. Skodol y D.S. Bender (Eds.), *Tratado de los trastornos de la personalidad* (pp. 17-36). Barcelona: Elsevier Masson.

Henry, C., Mitropoulou, V., New A.S., Koenigsberg, H.W., Silverman, J., and Siever, L.J. (2001). Affective instability and impulsivity in borderline personality and bipolar II disorders: similarities and differences. *Journal of Psychiatric Research,* 35, 307-312.

Kernberg, O.F. (1996). A psychoanalytic theory of personality disorders. In J.F. Clarkin, and M.F. Lenzenweger (Eds.), *Major theories on personality disorder* (pp.106-140). New York: Guilford Press.

Klosko, J. and Young, J. (2004).Cognitive therapy of borderline personality disorder. In R.L. Leahy (Ed.), *Contemporary cognitive therapy: theory, research and practice* (pp.269-299). New York: Guilford Press

Komarovskaya, I., Loper, A.B., and Warren, J. (2007). The role of impulsivity in antisocial and violent behavior and personality disorders among incarcerated women. *Criminal Justice and Behavior,* 34, 1499-1515.

Kremers, I.P., Spinhoven, P., Van der Does, A.J.W. (2004). Autobiographical memory in depressed and non-depressed patients with borderline personality disorder. *British Journal of Clinical Psychology*, 43, 17-29

Kremers, I.P., Van Giezen, A.E., Van der Does, A.M., Van Dyck, R., and Spinhoven, P. (2007). Memory of childhood trauma before and after long-term psychological treatment of borderline personality disorder. *Journal of Behavior Therapy and Experimental Psychiatry*, 38, 1-10

Krueger, R.F. (2005). Continuity of Axes I and II: toward a unified model of personality, personality disorders, and clinical disorders. *Journal of Personality Disorders,* 19, 233-261.

Lacey, J.H. and Evans, C.D. (1986). The impulsivist: a multi impulsive personality disorder. *British Journal of Addiction,* 81, 641-649.

Lara, D.R., Pinto, O., Akiskal, K., and Akiskal, H.S. (2006). Toward an integrative model of the spectrum of mood, behavioral and personality disorders based on fear and anger traits: I, clinical implications. *Journal of Affective Disorders,* 94, 67-87.

Lewis, M.D. (2000). Emotional self-organization at three time scales. In M.D. Lewis e I. Granic (Eds.), *Emotion, development and self-organization: Dynamic systems approaches to emotional development* (pp. 37-69). Cambridge, UK: Cambridge University Press.

Lineham, M.M. (1993b). *Skills training manual for treating borderline personality disorder.* New York: Guilford Press

Linehan, M.M. (1993a). *Cognitive-behavioral treatment of borderline personality disorder.* New York: Guilford Press.

Linehan, M.M., Armstrong, H.E., Suarez, A., et al. (1991). Cognitive-behavioral treatment of chronically parasuicidal borderline patients. *Archives of General Psychiatry,* 48, 1060-1064.

Linehan, M.M., Bohus, M., and Lynch, T.R. (2007).Dialectical Behavior Therapy for pervasive emotion dysregulation. In J.J. Gross (Ed.), *Handbook of emotion regulation* (pp. 581-605). New York: Guilford Press.

Linehan, M.M., Heard, H.L., and Armstrong, H.E. (1993). Naturalistic folow-up of a behavioral treatment for chronically parasuididal borderline patients. *Archives of General Psychiatry,* 50, 971-975.

Linehan, M.M., Tutek, D., Heard, H.L., et al. (1994). Interpersonal out-come of cognitive-behavioral treatment for chronically suicidal borderline patients. *American Journal of Psychiatry,* 5, 1771-1776.

Livesley, W.J. (2003). Diagnostic dilemmas in classifying personality disorder. In K.A. Phillips, M.B. First and H.A. Pincus (Eds.), Advancing *DSM: Dilemmas in psychiatric diagnosis* (pp. 153-190). Washington, DC: APA.

Livesley, W.J., and Jackson, D.N. (1999). Dimensional Assessment of Personality Pathology Manual. Port Huron: Sigma.

Lynam, D.R. and Widiger, T.A. (2001). Using the five-factor model to represent the DSM-IV personality disorders: an expert consensus approach. *Journal of Abnormal Psychology,* 110, 401-412.

Magai, C. and Hunziker, J. (1998). "To bedlam and part way back". Discrete emotions theory and borderline symptoms. In W.F. Flack and J.D. Laird (Eds.), *Emotions in Psychopatholoy* (pp. 380-393). New York: Oxford Press.

McClure, MM, Romero, MJ, Bowie, CR, Reichenberg, A, Harvey, PD, Siever, LJ (2007). Visual-spatial learning and memory in schizotypal personality disorder: Continued evidence for the importance of working memory in the schizophrenia spectrum. *Archives of Clinical Neuropsychology,* 22, 109-116.

Miller, J.D., Reynolds, S.K., and Pilkonis, P.A. (2004). The validity of the Five-Factor Model prototypes for personality disorders in two clinical samples. *Psychological Assessment,* 16, 310-322.

Millon, T. (1985). *Personality disorders: a biosocial learning approach.* New York: Wiley.

Millon, T. (1990). *Toward a new personology: an evolutionary model.* New York: Wiley-Interscience.

Millon, T. (2002). Assessment is not enough: the SPA should partipate in constructing a comprehensive clinical science of personality. *Journal of Personality Assessment,* 78, 209-218.

Minzenberg, M.J., Fisher-Irving, M., Poole, J.H., Vinogradov, S. (2006). Reduced self-referential source memory performance is associated with interpersonal dysfunction in borderline personality disorder. *Journal of Personality Disorders,* 20, 42-54

Mitropoulou, V., Harvey, P.D., Zegarelli, G., New, A.S., Silverman, J.M., and Siever, L.J. (2005). Neuropsychological performance in schizotypal personalitydisorder: Importance of working memory. *American Journal of Psychiatry,* 162, 1896-1903.

Morey, L.C. and Zanarini, M.D. (2000). Borderline personality: traits and disorder. *Journal of Abnormal Psychology,* 109, 733-737.

Muro, C., Tomas, C., Moreno, L., Rubio, V. (2002). Perception of aggression, personality disorders and psychiatric morbidity in nursing students. *Acta Psychiatrica Scandinavica,* 106, 118-120.

O`Connor, B.P. (2002). The search for dimensional structure differences between normality and abnormality: a statistical review of published data on personality and psychopathology. *Journal of Personality and Social Psychology,* 83, 962-982.

O`Connor, B.P. (2005). A search of consensus on the dimensional structure of personality disorders. *Journal of Clinical Psychology,* 61, 323-345.

Olivencia, J.J. y Cangas, A.J. (2002).Trastornos de personalidad. In A.J. Cangas, A.L. Maldonado and M. López (Eds.), *Manual de psicología clínica y general: vol. II Sicopatología* (pp.133-169). Granada: Alborán.

Paris, J. (1996). *Social factors in the personality disorders.* Cambridge: Cambridge University Press.

Pérez-Nieto, M.A., González Ordi, H. and Redondo, M.M. (2007). Procesos básicos en una aproximación cognitivo-conductual a los trastornos de personalidad. *Clínica y Salud,* 18, 401-423

Pérez-Nieto, M.A., Redondo, M.M. and Martín, M. (2004). Relaciones entre metacognición y control cognitivo e implicaciones en el ámbito de la psicopatología. *Edupsykhé,* 4, 233-250.

Pérez-Nieto, M.A., Redondo, M.M., Sánchez Burón, A. and Fernández, P. (in press). Implicaciones de la impulsividad y las creencias metacognitivas en el uso de estrategias de control cognitivo. In I. Etxebarria, A. Aritzeta, E. Barberá, M. Chóliz, M. P. Jiménez, F. Martínez, P. M. Mateos and D. Páez (Eds.), *Emoción y motivación: Contribuciones actuales* (Vol. II). Madrid: Asociación de Motivación y Emoción.

Porges, S. (1995). Orienting in a defensive world: mammalian modifications of our evolutionary heritage. A Polyvagal theory. *Psychophysiology, 32,* 301–318

Pretzer, J. and Beck, J.S. (2004). Cognitive therapy of personality disorders: twenty years of progress. In R.L. Leahy (Ed.), *Contemporary cognitive therapy: Theory, research and practice* (pp. 299-318). New York: Guilford Press.

Prieto, M, Vera, M.N., Pérez Marfil, MN, and Ramírez, I. (2007). Cronicidad de los trastornos del estado de ánimo: relaciones con actitudes cognitivas disfuncionales y con alteraciones de la personalidad. *Clínica y Salud,* 18, 203-219.

Quiroga Romero, E. and Errasti Pérez, J.M. (2001). Tratamientos psicológicos eficaces para los trastornos de personalidad. *Psicothema,* 13, 393-406.

Reitz, S., Krause-Utz,.A., Pogatzki-Zahn, EM, Ebner-Priemer, U., Bohus,M. and Schmahl, C. (2012). Stress Regulation and Incision in Borderline Personality Disorder—A Pilot Study Modeling Cutting Behavior. *Journal of Personality Disorders,* 26, 605-615.

Retz, W., Retz-Jnginger, P., Supprian, T., Thome, J. and Rosler, M. (2004). Association of serotonin transporter promoter gene polymorphism with violence: relation with personality disorders, impulsivity and childhood ADHD psychopathology. *Behavioral Sciences and The Law,* 22, 415-425.

Robins, C.J. (2002). Zen principles and mindfulness practice in dialectical behavior therapy. *Cognitive Behavioral Practice,* 9, 50-57.

Saulsman, L.M. and Page, A.C. (2004). The five-factor model and personality disorder empirical literature: A meta-analytic review. *Clinical Psychology Review,* 23, 1055-1085.

Schmahl, C., Meinzer, M., Zeuch, A., Fichter, M., Cebulla, M., Kleindienst, N., Ludäscher, P., Steil, R., and Bohus, M. (2012). Pain sensitivity is reduced in borderline personality disorder, but not in posttraumatic stress disorder and bulimia nervosa. *World Journal of Biological Psychiatry,* 11, 364-371.

Schmidt, N.B., Joiner, T.E., Young, J.E., et al. (1995). The Schema Questionnaire: investigation of psychometric properties and the hierarchical structure of a measure of maladaptative schemata. *Cognitve Therapy and Research,* 19, 295-321.

Schnell, K., Dietrich, T., Schnitker, R., Daumann, J., and Herpertz, S.C. (2007). Processing of autobiographical memory retrieval cues in borderline personality disorder. *Journal Of Affective Disorders,* 97, 253-259.

Segal, Z. (1988). Appraisal of the self schema: construct in cognitive models of depression. *Psychological Bulletin,* 103, 147-162.

Sherin, E.N., and Linehan, M.M. (1992). Patient-therapist ratings and relationship to progress in dialectical behavior therapy for borderline personality disorder. *Behaviour Therapy,* 23, 730-741.

Sieswerda, S., Arntz, A. and Kindt, M. (2007).Successful psychotherapy reduces hypervigilance in borderline personality disorder. *Behavioral and Cognitive Psychotherapy,* 35, 387-402.

Sieswerda, S., Arntz, A., Mertens, I. and Vertommen, S. (2007). Hypervigilance in patients with borderline personality disorder: Specificity, automaticity, and predictors. *Behavior Research and Therapy,* 45, 1011-1024.

Silbersweig, D., Clarkin, J.F., Goldstein, M., Kernberg, O.F., Tuescher, O., and Levy, K.N. (2007). Failure of frontolimbic inhibitory function in the context of negative emotion in borderline personality disorder. *American Journal of Psychiatry,* 164, 1832-1841.

Skodol, A.E., Gunderson, J.G., Shea, M.T., McGlashan, T.H.., Morey, L.C., et al. (2005). The collaborative Longitudinal Personality disorders Study (CLPS). *Journal of Personality Disorder,* 19, 487-504.

Stanley, B. and Brodsky, B.S. (2007).Terapia dialéctica conductual. In J.M. Oldham, A.E. Skodol y D.S. Bender (Eds.), *Tratado de los trastornos de la personalidad* (pp. 309-322). Barcelona: Elsevier Masson.

Stevens, A., Burkhardt, M., Hautzinger, M., Schwarz, J., and Unckel, C. (2004). Borderline personality disorder: impaired visual perception and working memory. *Psychiatric Research,* 125, 257-267.

Svrakic, D.M., Draganic, S., Hill, K., et al. (2002). Temperament, character, and personality disorders: etiologic, diagnostic and treatment issues. *Acta Psychiatrica Scandinavica,* 106, 189-195.

Szerman, N. (2004).Impulsividad y trastornos de personalidad. In S. Ros Montalbán, M.D. Peris Díaz and R. Gracia Marco (Eds.), *Impulsividad* (pp. 101-119). Barcelona: Ars Medica.

Trull, T.J. and Durrett, C.A. (2005).Categorical and dimensional models of personality disorder. *Annual Review of Clinical Psychology,*1, 355-380.

Trull, T.J., Widiger, T.A., Lynam, D.R., et al. (2003). Borderline personality disorder from the perspective of general personality functioning. *Journal of Abnormal Psychology,* 112, 193-202.

Turkat, I.D. and Maisto, S.A. (1985). Personality disorders: Application of the experimental method to the formulation and modification of personality disorders. In D.H. Barlow (Ed.), *Clinical handbook of psychological disorders: A step by step treatment manua*l. New York: Guilford Press.

Tyrer, P., Coombs, N., Ibrahimi, F., Mathilakath, A., Bajaj, P., et al. (2007). Critical developments in the assessment of personality disorder. *British Journal of Psychiatry, Suppl.,* 49, 51-59.

Valenzuela, J. and Caballo, V.E. (2001). La terapia de esquemas, de Young. In V.E. Caballo (Ed.), *Manual de los trastornos de personalidad: descripción, evaluación y tratamiento* (pp. 463-481). Madrid: Síntesis.

Watson, D., and Tellegen, A. (1985). Toward a consensual structure of mood. *Psychological Bulletin,* 98, 219-235.

Wells, A. (2000). *Emotional Disorders and Metacognition: Innovative Cognitive Therapy*. Chichester: Wiley.

Widiger, T.A. and Costa, P.T. (2002). Five factor model personality disorder research. In P.T. Costa and Widiger, T.A. (Eds.), *Personality disorders and the Five Factor Model of Personality, 2nd Edition* (pp.59-87). Washington, DC: American Psychological Association.

Widiger, T.A. and Mullins-Sweatt, M.A. (2007).Modelos categoriales y dimensionales de los trastornos de personalidad. In J.M. Oldham, A.E. Skodol and D.S. Bender (Eds.), *Tratado de los trastornos de la personalidad* (pp. 37-55). Barcelona: Elsevier Masson.

Widiger, T.A. and Samuel, D.B. (2005).Diagnostic categories or dimensions? A question for the Diagnostic *and Statistical Manual of Mental Disorders –Fifth Edition. Journal of Abnormal Psychology,* 114, 494-504.

Williams, L.M., Sidis, A., Gordon, E., Meares, R.A. (2006). "Missing links" in borderline personality disorder: loss of neural synchrony relates to lack of emotion regulation and impulse control. *Journal of Psychiatry and Neuroscience,* 31, 181-188.

Wingenfeld, K., Mensebach, C, Rullkoetter, N., et al. (2009). Attentional Bias to Personally Relevant Words in Borderline Personality Disorder is Strongly Related to Comorbid Posttraumatic Stress Disorder. *Journal of Personality Disorders,* 23, 141-155.

Young, J.E. (1999). *Cognitive therapy for personality disorders*. Sarasota, FL: Professional Resources Press.

Young, J.E. and Klosko, J. (2007).Terapia de esquemas. In J.M. Oldham, A.E. Skodol and D.S. Bender (Eds.), *Tratado de los trastornos de la personalidad* (pp. 289-308). Barcelona: Elsevier Masson.

Young, J.E., Klosko, J.S. and Weishaar, M.E. (2003). *Schema therapy: a practitioner's guide*. New York: Guilford Press.

In: Mental Health and Psychiatry ISBN: 978-1-62417-589-3
Editors: A.S. Wilson and M.S. Schneider

Chapter 2

SENSORY IMPAIRMENT AND MENTAL HEALTH

Jesper Dammeyer* and Ola Hendar
University of Copenhagen, Department of Psychology, Copenhagen, Denmark

ABSTRACT

Sensory impairment - hearing impairment, visual impairment or deaf-blindness - is found to increase the risk of developing mental health problems of almost all kinds. The aim of this chapter is to present and discuss research findings concerning the associations between sensory impairment and mental health. Focus will be on two different explanations: First, common genetic or neurological components may cause both sensory impairment and mental health problems. Second that sensory impairment affects communicative abilities, social interaction, and limits input from the surrounding environment, all of which may increase the individual's level of stress in everyday life.

Research in correlation between sensory impairment and mental health issues is important both in order to better understand the impact of sensory impairment on human functioning and to gain more knowledge about mental health and sensation in general.

The chapter starts with a review of existing research regarding the prevalence of mental health problems in persons with visual impairment,

* Corresponding address: Jesper Dammeyer, University of Copenhagen, Department of Psychology, Øster Farimagsgade 2A, 1353 København K, Jesper.dammeyer@psy.ku.dk, jesper@dammeyer.dk, phone 0045+22808389.

hearing impairment, and dual sensory loss, respectively. Mental health issues of special interest will be elaborated upon according to type of sensory impairment, for example cases of depression among elderly people with acquired deaf-blindness and cases of autism among children with congenital blindness. A major topic will be discussions of how communication and language difficulties following sensory impairment are associated with mental health problems. For children, in particular, sensory impairment may result in language delays that may have serious consequences for their development. Finally, clinical issues will be discussed, for example challenges regarding assessment, differential diagnostics, and recommended treatment procedures.

In conclusion, sensory impairment, in most cases, is not a direct cause to mental health problems but is a contributing factor to an increased vulnerability towards developing mental health disorders. Communication and language development are found to be one of the most important components in prevention and treatment of mental health problems among individuals with sensory impairment.

Keywords: Blindness; Deafness; Deaf-blindness; Dual sensory impairment; Communication; Hearing impairment; Mental health; Psychiatry; Sensory impairment; Visual impairment

Epidemiological Findings of Mental Health Problems among Individuals with Sensory Impairment

To understand associations between sensory impairment and mental health, it would be advantageous to start with information about prevalence. In the following, we review existing research of the prevalence of mental health problems among individuals with hearing impairment, visual impairment, and deaf-blindness (dual sensory loss), respectively. First we will give a short introduction to the etiology of sensory impairment and the differences between congenital and acquired sensory impairment.

Etiology of Sensory Impairment

Etiology of visual impairment, hearing impairment and deaf-blindness include hereditary, pre- peri- and postnatal causes and a number of diseases throughout the lifespan. Heterogenic causes include a large number of genetic syndromes. The Pendred syndrome (causes congenital hearing impairment) and the Usher syndrome (may cause both vision and hearing impairment) just to mention a few. Prenatal causes include infections of the fetus, e.g. Rubella virus infection or Cytomegalovirus, which both may cause vision and hearing impairment. Perinatal causes are for example low birth weight, which is found to be one of the major causes of congenital blindness (Mervis, Yargin-Allsopp, Winter, and Boyle, 2000). Postnatal causes include injuries, blindness following diabetes, intoxications etc. In old age, the major causes to vision impairment are age-related macular degeneration, cataracts, and glaucoma (Klaver, Wolfs, Vingerling, Hofman, and de Jong, 1998) and to hearing impairment presbycusis, (i.e. age-related sensorineural hearing loss) (van Eyken, Camp, and Laer, 2007).

The number of cases with unknown etiology has been reported as being approximately 25% among individuals with congenital deaf-blindness (Dammeyer, 2010c) and hearing impairment (Korver et al., 2011) and approximately 9% among individuals with visual impairment (Blohmé, Bengtsson-Stigmar, and Tornqvist, 2000).

Congenital or Acquired Sensory Impairment

People with congenital sensory impairment are either born deaf and/or blind or become deaf and/or blind during the first stages of life before the development of language (pre-lingual sensory impairment). Post-lingual sensory impairment refers to people who become deaf and/or blind after the development of language (acquired sensory impairment). The consequences are significantly different depending on whether the sensory impairment is congenital or acquired. Congenital sensory impairment presents challenging conditions for language acquisition and learning an alternative language mode (congenital deaf children may use sign-language) becomes necessary. As explained later, congenital sensory impairment has in general a great notable effect on cognitive and social development.

Visual Impairment and Mental Health

The overall prevalence of visual impairment is approximately 1:1000 (Blohmé et al., 2000). Congenital blindness is often accompanied by additional disabilities, e.g. cerebral palsy, seizure disorders or developmental disabilities. In a study of 228 visually impaired children in metropolitan Atlanta between 1991 and 1993, 154 (68%) had an additional disability (Mervis et al., 2000). Neurological damages may affect both visual perception, other cognitive abilities (Blohmé et al., 2000), and cause mental and behavioral disorders.

Congenital visual impairment alone can have a variety of impacts on development: Cognitive, motor, emotional, communicative development among others (Warren and Hatton, 2003). The child's visual impairment may first of all have an impact on both the child and the caregiver's abilities to engage in social interaction and communication from early in life. Vision is the basis for prelinguistic communication characterized by face-to-face orientation and eye-to-eye contact (Preisler, 1991). The challenges in pre-linguistic communication impact considerably other aspects of the child's development (Warren and Hatton, 2003) including mental health.

One of the consequences of early difficulties in pre-linguistic communication seems to be symptoms of autism spectrum disorder (Hobson and Bishop, 2003). Autism, or autism-related conditions, is common among congenitally blind children (Cass, 1998; Mukaddes et al., 2007), almost half of children between 3 and 9 years has been found to meet the formal diagnostic criteria for autism (Brown et al., 1997). (See the section "Theory of Mind" for a further discussion of the association of sensory impairment and symptoms of autism spectrum disorder.).

Mental health problems have also been identified among individuals with acquired visual impairment. Visual impairment is a strong predictor for depression. Depression and anxiety are therefore consistently reported as being associated with visual impairment (Bazargan and Hamm-Baugh, 1995). Moreover, Lam, Christ, Lee, Zheng and Arheart (2008) reported a higher risk of suicide among people with a visual impairment.

Lam et al (2008) described other consequences associated with visual impairments such as social isolation, cognitive impairment, and functional decline. With a visual impairment, it may be difficult to maintain daily routines and mobility. This increases the likelihood of social withdrawal, and isolation which may affect the individual's quality of life. Research has documented that individuals who underwent cataract surgery experienced significant improvements in their quality of life, in addition to improved vision (Owsley et al., 2007). Social support has been found to be an important factor for individuals with vision impairment. High quality social support correlates for example with fewer depressive symptoms (Reinhardt, 1996).

Hearing Impairment

Prevalence of congenital deafness has been reported to be around 3:1000 (van Naarden, 1999; Watkin and Baldwin, 2011). As with children with visual impairment, deafness is often coupled with additional disabilities. Additional disabilities have been reported in around 20-30% of the population of children with congenital hearing impairment (Fellinger, Holzinger, and Polland, 2012; Hendar, 2008; 2012; Dammeyer, 2010a; Hindley, 2005). Additional neurodevelopmental problems have been reported in 30% and intellectual disabilities in 26% of children in a group with hearing impairment (van Naarden, Decouflé, and Caldwall, 1999).

Deafness and hearing impairment may affect both language, social and cognitive development (Mayberry, 2003). Several research reports around the world have documented a higher prevalence of all aspects of mental health problems among both children and adults with hearing impairment. The National Institute for Mental Health in England reported a prevalence of 40% of mental health problems among deaf children where the prevalence among children without hearing impairment was only 25%. (National Institute for mental Health, 2005). Two other examples are surveys from Sweden and Norway which report a higher prevalence of general mental health symptoms, anxiety and depression among deaf adults compared to adults without hearing impairments (Tambs, 2004, Kvam, 2006; Werngren-Elgström et al., 2003). In Norway, Kvam (2006) collected information using a symptom checklist among 431 deaf persons from different age-spans. Werngren-Elgström and colleagues (2003) collected data from a group of elderly pre-lingual deaf persons using sign-language.

Fellinger et al. (2012) reported in a review that deafness has far reaching consequences on social, emotional and cognitive development. There have been many occurrences of autism found within the group of children with hearing loss (Carvill, 2001; Jure, Rapin, and Tuchman, 1991), and similar to children with visual impairment, early language and communicative difficulties may explain part of the symptoms observed. (See the section "Theory of Mind" for an elaborated discussion of this issue).

Deaf Blindness

Deaf-blindness – i.e. dual sensory impairment – refers to the co-existence of both visual and hearing impairment. While congenital deaf-blindness is a rare condition (Dammeyer, 2010c) acquired deaf-blindness is frequent among elderly people. Where prevalence was close to 0% among adults below 65 years old, prevalence rose to 27% among individuals above 80 years of age (Schneider et al., 2012). Severe mental and behavioral disorders have been reported to be common among individuals with congenital deaf-blindness. Dammeyer (2011) found that among 95 adults with congenital deaf-blindness, 74% did have a mental and/or behavioral disorder. Mental retardation was found among 34%, psychosis among 13%, autism among 2%, mood disorder among 11%, obsessive-compulsive disorder among 5%, anxiety disorder among 4%, and behavioral disorder (e.g. hyperactivity and/or conduct disorder) among 5%. A higher prevalence of mental and behavioral disorders is also found among people with acquired deaf-blindness. Studies have found an increased risk of depression (Chou and Chi, 2004; Capella-McDonalld, 2005; Lupsakko, Mantyjarvi, Kautiainen, and Sulkava, 2002) among elderly people with dual sensory loss compared to individuals without sensory impairment, but also compared to individuals with vision or hearing loss alone. Deaf-blindness among elderly has also been found to be associated with poor self-rated health and decreased participation in social activities. People with dual sensory loss were for example found to have approximately 10% lower rates of participation in activities such as visiting friends (Crews and Campbell, 2004). Cognitive decline among people with acquired deaf-blindness may be seen as a result of the interaction between dual sensory loss and mental and behavioral disorders. Laforge, Spector, and Sternberg (1992) found, after adjusting for age, sex and cognitive status, that persons who had a visual impairment or both a vision and a hearing impairment were 2.5 and 3.5 times more likely to experience functional decline than were unimpaired older adults, respectively. In a large study of 6112 women aged 69 and older, Lin et al. (2004) found similar odds for reduced cognitive function (2.19) for women with combined visual and hearing impairment as compared to women without impairments. The above sections demonstrate that all kinds of mental health problems occur across all groups of individuals with sensory impairments. In the following sections the aim is to discuss why this higher prevalence is found.

Communication, Communication, Communication

Overall, the same conclusion is made in several studies of sensory impairment and mental health: Communication development or communication rehabilitation is one of the most important issues in preventing mental health difficulties. In the following sections we will discuss some of these studies.

Congenital Deaf Children and Psychosocial Wellbeing

To pick out one example among children with congenital deafness, Dammeyer (2010a) studied 334 Danish children in order to assess their psychosocial wellbeing and to find explaining variables. Overall, the study found a prevalence of psychosocial problems that were almost four times as large compared to a group of hearing children. It was found that the child's communicative skills, either oral or signed, determined whether the children experienced psychosocial difficulties or not. If the child's spoken or sign language abilities were sufficient (i.e. were able to communicate without difficulties) no higher incidence of psychosocial problems was found.

Differing from the children's communicative abilities (regardless of communication modality) being a key factor, the degree of hearing loss (deaf or hearing impairment) had no impact on the child's psychosocial wellbeing. It thus appears that hearing impairment itself is not a direct cause of a child's low psychosocial well-being, rather it is how well the child is able to succeed in linguistic/communicative development that is essential. The same results have been reported in other international studies, for example in a study by Stevenson and colleagues (2010) in England. Fellinger and colleagues (2012) state in an overview of mental health and children with hearing impairment, that "*language and communication environment of the family is a crucial variable affecting psychosocial wellbeing of deaf children*". (Fellinger et al., 2012, p. 1039).

Dual Sensory Loss and Communication

Similar findings, demonstrating association between communication and mental health, appear among individuals with dual sensory loss. McDonneall (2009) found that communication and social support were important to avoid the experience of depression among people with acquired deaf-blindness. A similar pattern is evident among adults with congenital deaf-blindness. Dammeyer (2010d) found a strong association between low communication abilities and low cognitive functioning among people with congenital deaf-blindness, indicating an interrelation between dual sensory loss, cognitive function and communication.

Visual Impairment and Communication

As already introduced, communication may also be a crucial issue for children with congenital blindness (Preisler, 1991), where early communicative difficulties may lead to both cognitive and social difficulties (Warren and Hatteon, 2003). Studies have demonstrated that the inability to share perspectives and attention with others interferes with language and cognitive development in young children with visual impairment (Bigelow, 1990).

SPECIFIC SYNDROMES AND BIOLOGICAL CAUSES

Specific syndromes which include sensory impairment have been presumed to be associated with a higher prevalence of some specific mental and behavioral disorders. In the following, we will discuss two syndromes: Usher syndrome and Congenital Rubella syndrome. The overall question in this section is: To what degree is the observed increased risk of mental health problems caused by biological damages linked to specific syndromes which also include sensory impairment?

Usher Syndrome

Usher syndrome is characterized by deafness and a gradual loss of vision. The hearing loss is sensorineural, whereas the vision loss is associated with retinitis pigmentosa (RP), which is a degeneration of the retinal cells, leading to increased tunnel vision. The hearing impairment is congenital and profound in some types of Usher syndrome and moderate in other types. Different mental and behavioral disorders have been reported among adults. Hallgren (1959) reported that 23% of 114 individuals with Usher syndrome were psychotic and Nuutila (1970) reported a prevalence of 4.5% among 133 individuals. Psychosis has also been reported in a number of case studies (Mangotich and Misiaszek, 1983; Hess-Röver, Crichton and Holland, 1999; Jumaian and Fergusson, 2003; McDonald, Kenna and Larkin, 1998; Viala,

Nicot, Levy and Vacheron, 2009; Koizumi, 1988; Wu and Chiu, 2006; Rais, 2006). Mental retardation (Sharp et al., 1994), anorexia nervosa (Chapman, Valmana, and Lacey, 1998) and ADHD (Rijavec and Grubic, 2009) have also been reported occurring among individuals with Usher syndrome. Stress, anxiety, social isolation and depression are other mental health related issues that are proposed to be associated with Usher syndrome (Miner, 1995; Damen, Krabbe, Kilsby, and Mylanus, 2005).

In a recent study of 26 children with Usher syndrome (Dammeyer, 2012a), 6 were found to be diagnosed with a mental or behavioral disorder (1 with schizophrenia and mild mental retardation, 1 with atypical autism and severe mental retardation, 1 with atypical autism and mild mental retardation, 1 with mild mental retardation, and 2 with conduct disorder). Another 3 children had had a mental or behavioral disorder previously in their childhood. Among the children without any current mental or behavioral disorders, 5 (27%) experienced psychosocial difficulties. (Psychosocial difficulties were not assessed among children with a current mental or behavioral disorder.) All together, more than 40% of the children with Usher syndrome were found to have mental health problems.

Two explanations for a higher incidence of mental health problems among children and adults with Usher syndrome are discussed. Some researchers argue that the progressive loss of vision results in severe stress that leads to symptoms of mental and/or behavioral disorders. Case studies report that mental and behavioral symptoms in patients with Usher syndrome develop simultaneously with the loss of vision (Mangotich and Misiaszek, 1983; Rais, 2006; Hallgren, 1959). Severe communicative difficulties, following the loss of vision, may be a major source of the experienced stress.

The second possible explanation for an association between Usher syndrome and mental and behavioral disorders is that some genes are predisposed to both Usher syndrome and for example schizophrenia (McDonald et al., 1998). Studies of families with more than one member with Usher syndrome and schizophrenia support this hypothesis (Wu and Chiu, 2006; Sharp et al., 1994; Karjalainen, Teräsvirta, Kärjä, and Kääriäinen, 1983). However, until now no specific genes or mutations have been reported as being possible candidates. Mental and behavioral disorders may be a consequence of brain abnormalities associated with Usher syndrome (McDonald et al., 1998). Schaefer and colleagues (Schaefer, 1998) found that the measured volume of the brain was significantly smaller compared to normal controls and Koizumi et al. (1988) found a global degeneration of the brain in one case with Usher syndrome and schizophrenia.

Contradicting the genetic explanation of mental and behavioral disorders is the fact that only some individuals with Usher syndrome are found to have mental health problems and the nomenclature of difficulties is not uniform. Either different Usher genes are associated with different kinds of mental health problems, or severe stress and communicative difficulties are related to the sensory impairment.

Congenital Rubella Syndrome

Another example is individuals with Congenital Rubella Syndrome (CRS). Rubella infection contracted by a woman in the early stages of pregnancy may cause serious health problems for the affected fetus. From birth, the baby may experience mild to severe sensorineural hearing loss, cataracts, cardiac problems, and damages to the brain and nervous system (Duszak, 2009; Webster, 1998). Mental and behavioral disorders have been suggested as specific delayed manifestations of the Rubella infection. Progressive rubella panencephalitis (PRP) has been proposed (Sever, South, and Shaver, 1985) as a possible name for a slowly progressive and fatal disease of the central nervous system that is caused by the chronic Rubella virus infection of the brain. Twelve cases have been reported (Waxham and Wolinsky, 1984). Symptoms of PRP have commonly been observed developing in the second decade of life (Sever et al., 1985) and may include learning problems, ataxia and cognitive decline with progression to seizures, cerebral palsy, and psychosis. Behavior problems, anxiety attacks, anger, crying and self-injury and other mental health problems have also been reported as possible consequences of CRS (O'Donnell, 1991). The question is whether these observed mental health problems are solely the consequence of the Rubella virus or may also be associated with congenital sensory impairment.

In a study of 35 congenitally deafblind individuals with CRS (Dammeyer, 2010b), no specific incidence of mental and behavioral disorders could be found. None of the specific PRP symptoms or other delayed manifestation could be confirmed when the individuals with CRS were compared to a control group of individuals who were congenitally deafblind with different etiology than CRS. The study concludes that the mental health related problems which people with CRS face are primarily a consequence of the congenital deaf-blindness and language deprivation.

The two examples, Usher and Rubella syndrome, show that a common neurological, genetic or chromosomal disorder may in some cases cause both sensory impairment and mental and behavioral disorders, but often a more complex association between different factors is the case. Here communication abilities and language development play a significant part. Therefore, it is important to determine the pattern of factors affecting the person in each particular case.

EXPLORING ASSOCIATIONS BETWEEN LANGUAGE DEVELOPMENT AND MENTAL HEALTH PROBLEMS: COCHLEA IMPLANT, SIGN LANGUAGE AND THEORY OF MIND

The following sections elaborate on selected issues illustrating the associations between sensory impairment and mental health problems. Again, language and communicative development is the main focus in the following examples.

Cochlear Implantation

In the past decade, debates have focused on how deaf children's use of cochlear implants (CI) may improve mental health conditions (Bat-Chava, Martin, and Kosciw, 2005; Boyd, Knutson, and Dahlstrom, 2000; Huber, 2005; Khan, Edwards, and Langdon, 2005; Nicholas and Geers, 2003). Studies find that CI improves the overall mental health condition of children with congenital hearing impairment.

However, studies controlling for multiple variables, including additional disabilities and sign-language abilities, do not find that CI alone improves mental health among children with congenital hearing impairment (for example Dammeyer, 2010a).

These studies conclude that early communicative development is the overall most important issue, not type of hearing aid, mode of communication (signed or oral) or degree of hearing loss. Nevertheless, CI and other types of hearing aids (and similar visual aids for children with visual impairment), contribute positively towards mental health condition, if the aid support communicative functioning and language development.

Sign-Language

Controversies between a medical/audiological versus a cultural/ecological perspective on deafness (Blume, 1999; Hindley et al., 1994; Polat, 2003) are part of the debates about mental health problems among children with hearing impairment. A bicultural and bilingual perspective has been found to contribute to deaf children's communicative, social and cognitive development because it gives the children a greater ability to communicate from early in life and an ability to develop a self-image and self-esteem as a deaf person (Heiling, 1995; Hindley, 2000). Studies also find that sign language abilities correlate with psychosocial well-being (Polat, 2003; Sinkkonen, 1994; Stevenson et al., 2010; Dammeyer, 2010a). Parental hearing status has also been discussed as an important factor within this perspective (Mayberry, 2003) where for example Polat (2003) found that deaf children of deaf parents had a better psychosocial adjustment than deaf children of hearing parents.

Even though it has been found that mode of language in itself does not make a difference to the level of experienced mental health problems, some cultural language influence may still be important. Sign language is a minority language with the same prerequisites as any other minority language. Sign language and sign-language users may meet cultural barriers in society at large and even suppression (Ladd, 2003, Reagan 2010). Risks of cultural stress and marginalization are present being part of a minority culture and using a minority language and this may explain some of the mental health problems people with hearing loss experience.

Theory of Mind Development

To illustrate the importance of early language acquisition among children with sensory impairment and the associations with mental health problems, development of Theory of Mind can be picked out as a good example. Theory of Mind is the ability to attribute mental states (beliefs, desires, etc.) to oneself and others and to understand that others have mental states that are different from one's own. Most researchers agree that the ability to exercise Theory of Mind does not develop before the age of 3-4 (Peterson, 2004). It has been suggested that Theory of Mind is important in social and cognitive development and delayed Theory of Mind development may be associated with a higher risk of mental health problems.

As already mentioned, congenitally blind children may experience difficulties in perspective taking and Theory of Mind. These problems are associated with the children's language and communicative difficulties (Warren and Hatton, 2003). A lot of research has also been conducted concerning how Theory of Mind development is affected by congenital hearing loss (Mayberry 2003, Peterson, 2004). Theory of mind abilities are often developed later among deaf children, which appears to be associated with the communicative difficulties these children experience. Deaf children, who grow up in a sign language environment, using sign language as their first language do not encounter delayed acquisition of Theory of Mind compared to hearing peers. However, deaf children who learn sign language at a later age often experience a delayed development of Theory of Mind abilities (Meristo et al., 2007; Peterson and Siegal, 1999). Therefore, it appears that the development of an efficient mode of communication early in life is a necessary prerequisite for well-developed Theory of Mind abilities.

The effect of early cochlear implantation has been investigated regarding its influence on Theory of Mind development. Peterson (2004) found that level of language development significantly predicted ability of Theory of Mind, but deaf children with cochlear implants were just as delayed in Theory of Mind development as their deaf peers with hearing aids. This study also concluded that regardless of mode of communication or level of hearing impairment early communication abilities were the important factor.

The above examples (cochlear implant, sign language and Theory of Mind development) all illustrate how congenital sensory impairment may have a notable and complex impact on psychological and mental health development. However, the examples also illustrate that it is possible to prevent and possibly eliminate most of the consequences of sensory impairment. Next section will concern clinical assessment and intervention issues.

Clinical Assessment and Intervention

For patients with sensory impairment, as with all other patients affected by mental health problems, correct and effective diagnosis and treatment are important for any chance of assuring improvement. Individuals with sensory impairments may meet specific barriers within mental health services. For example, communication may be difficult since most professionals are not able to communicate using sign language or to understand aspects of the Deaf culture. Deaf patients report fear, mistrust, and frustrations in health care settings (Steinberg et al., 2006). The following sections discuss some of the issues that need to be addressed in clinical practice working with children and adults with sensory impairment.

Differential Diagnostics

Differentiating between symptoms of sensory impairment and symptoms of mental and behavioral disorder can be a difficult task. Diagnosing autism spectrum disorder is one example. The communicative, social and cognitive symptoms of autism may be similar to symptoms of dual sensory loss (Hoevenaars-van den Boom, Antonissen, Knoors, and Vervloed, 2009). Self-injurious (biting and hitting) or self-stimulating behavior (rocking, looking into light etc.) is often found in individuals with congenital deaf-blindness. The behavior can be interpreted as compensation for the lack of sensory input and/or as an expression of frustration because of the lack of language/communication skills (Hoevenaars-van den Boomet et al., 2009), and is different from the restricted, repetitive and stereotyped patterns of behavior seen in people with autism, psychosis and mental retardation.

The self-injurious behavior shown by congenitally deaf-blind children usually decreases when helpful progressive measures are taken, such as useful communication and/or vision and hearing aids (Janssen and Rødbroe, 2007). The risk of incorrect assessment and interpretation of behavior is over-diagnosis and/or inappropriate treatment of mental health problems in people with sensory impairment. Similarly, people with mental retardation have been undiagnosed for sensory impairment and therefore have not received appropriate treatment (Fellinger, Holzinger, Dirmhirn, van Dijk, and Goldberg, 2009; Meuwese-Jongejeugd et al., 2008), and are another example of the difficulties of detecting and differentiating between sensory impairment and mental health problems.

Like any other organic or somatic causes to mental and behavioral disorders, e.g. head trauma, tumor, drug abuse etc., vision and hearing impairments need to be checked and treated upon the first signs of mental health problems. Even for a person with severe developmental disabilities, it is vital to compensate for the sensory loss by introducing hearing and visual aids and communicative skills. Treatment of mental health problems among individuals with sensory impairment is in many cases a matter of progressing as far as possible with the development of the person's communicative abilities to reduce the negative impact of the sensory loss (Dammeyer, 2012b).

Assessment

It is generally difficult to use traditional psychological and psychiatric tests and diagnostic tools to assess mental health of persons with sensory loss since the assessment tools often require full sensory functioning as a prerequisite (Ronnberg and Borg, 2001). Therefore, it is important to triangulate diagnostic tools and procedures.

Both structured and non-structured observation, formal and informal tests must be applied. Diagnostic procedures of a patient with dual sensory loss and mental health problems often need to be a multiannual and cross-disciplinary task of speech and vision- and hearing therapists, psychologists, psychiatrists, physiotherapists, etc. with experience working with patients with sensory impairment and mental health problems.

It is important to continuously monitor and analyze the functioning of vision, hearing, and communicative abilities of the person in case. Video observation is a useful tool, which specifically can add value to some of the key parameters in relation to the relevant diagnose. Andersen and Rødbroe (2000), and Dammeyer (2012b) describe approaches of video observations of congenitally deafblind individuals that may also be useful for deaf and blind children with severe additional disabilities.

In the following sections we discuss how assessment of mental and behavioral disorders can be carried out in clinical practice.

Assessing Autism Spectrum Disorder

Many of the diagnostic tools used to diagnose autism are not compatible with the particular difficulties faced by individuals with deafblindness (Hoevenaars-van den Boom et al., 2009) and a standardized test is also problematic in the case of deaf (Edwards and Crocker, 2008) and blind children (Hobson and Bishop, 2003). A person with severe sensory impairment may seem uninterested in other persons, show abnormal behavior, and have severe communicative difficulties without having an autism spectrum disorder. In order to differentiate between autism and sensory disability, it is important to examine the person's social behavior in a familiar setting, for example the child together with a familiar grown-up communicative partner (Janssen and Rødbroe, 2007).

Assessing Cognitive Abilities

Even though a child with vision and/or hearing impairment has normal cognitive functioning, the sensory loss may give the child some functionally serious cognitive difficulties if the child's language development is delayed. The older the child gets, the more the child is at risk to ''fall behind'' as compared to a hearing and sighted child.

The sensory impaired child requires more time, as information does not reach the child all that easily. Some congenitally sensory impaired children – and adults - exhibit normal cognitive abilities, nevertheless, they do not function in accordance with their age.

It is not possible to use all cognitive tests on either deaf (Maller, 1997; Edwards and Crocker, 2008) or blind individuals (Warren and Hatton, 2003). Intellectual disability needs to be assessed by psychologists with experience in administering formal tests to persons with sensory impairment. Leiter-R (Roid and Miller, 1997) or another non-verbal instrument will in most cases be appropriate to apply on children with hearing impairments. On children with visual impairments, a non-visual test can be used with success, for example the IVIC (Intelligence test for Visually Impaired Children) (Dekker, Drenth, Zaal, and Koole, 1990).

Conclusion

The risk of developing mental health problems is overall higher among individuals with sensory impairment compared to individuals without sensory impairment. Two explanations co-exist: The same biological defect causes both sensory impairment and mental health problems.

An example is genetic syndromes which cause both intellectual disability and sensory impairment. The second explanation is that the higher risk of mental health problems can be attributed to the sensory impairment which leads to communicative and language difficulties, limited access to information and social participation. The focus in clinical assessment and rehabilitation practice needs to be, in addition to vision and hearing aids, on rehabilitation of communicative and social functioning. For children with congenital sensory impairment early intervention on language and communicative development is crucial.

REFERENCES

Andersen, K. and Rødbroe, I. (2000). *Identification of Congenital Deaf-blindness*. Aalborg, Denmark: The Danish Resource Centre on Congenital Deaf-blindness.

Bat-Chava, Y., Martin, D., and Kosciw, J. G. (2005). Longitudinal Improvements in Communication and Socialization of Deaf Children with Cochlear Implants and Hearing Aids: Evidence from Parental Reports. *Journal of Psychology and Psychiatry, 46*, 1287-1296.

Bazargan, M. and Hamm-Baugh, V. P. (1995). The Relationship Between Chronic Illness and Depression in a Community of Black Elderly Persons. *Journal of Gerontology: Social Sciences, 50B*(2), 119-127.

Bigelow, A. (1990). Relationship between the Development of Language and Thought in Young Blind Children. *Journal of Visual Impairment and Blindness, 84*(8), 414-419.

Blohmé, J., Bengtsson-Stigmar, E., and Tornqvist, K. (2000). Visually Impaired Swedish Children. Longitudinal comparisons 1980-1999. *Acta Ophthalmologica Scandinavica, 78,* 416-429.

Blume, S. B. (1999). Histories of Cochlear Implantation. *Social Science and Medicine, 49*, 1257-1268.

Boyd, R. C., Knutson, J. F., and Dahlstrom, A. J. (2000). Social Interaction of Pediatric Cochlear Implant Recipients with Age-Matched Peers. *Annals of Otology, Rhinology and Laryngology, 185(suppl.)*, 105-109.

Brown, R., Hobson, R. P., Lee, A. and Stevenson, J. (1997*).* Are There 'Autistic-Like' Features in Congenitally Blind Children? *Journal of Child Psychology and Psychiatry and Allied Disciplines, 38,* 693-703.

Capella-McDonnall, M. (2005). The effects of single and dual sensory loss on symptoms of depression in the elderly. *International Journal of Geriatric Psychiatry, 20*, 855-861.

Carvill, S. (2001). *Sensory* Impairments, Intellectual Disability and Psychiatry. *Journal of Intellectual Disability Research*, *47*(6), 467-483.

Cass, H. (1998). Visual Impairment and Autism. *Autism, 2(2)*, 117-138.

Chapman, V., Valmana, A., and Lacey, J. H. (1998). A Case Report of Usher's Syndrome and Anorexia Nervosa. *International Journal of Eating Disorder, 23*, 223-226.

Chou, K. and Chi, I. (2004). Combined effects of vision and hearing impairment on depression in elderly Chinese. *International Journal of Geriatric Psychiatry, 19*, 825-832.

Crews, J. E. and Campbell, V. A. (2004). Vision Impairment and Hearing Loss Among Community Dwelling Older Americans: Implications for Health and Functioning. American Journal of Public Health, 94*(5), 823-829.*

Damen, G. W. J. A., Krabbe, P. F. M., Kilsby, M., and Mylanus, E. A. M. (2005). The Usher Lifestyle Survey: Maintaining Independence: A Multi-Centre Study. *International Journal of Rehabilitation Research, 28*(4), 309-328.

Dammeyer, J. (2010a). Psychosocial Development in a Danish Population of Children with Cochlear Implants and Deaf and Hard of Hearing Children. *Journal of Deaf Studies and Deaf Education, 15*(1), 50-58.

Dammeyer, J. (2010b). Congenital Rubella Syndrome and Delayed Manifestations. International Journal of Pediatric Otorhinolaryngology, *74*(9), 1067-1070.

Dammeyer, J. (2010c). Prevalence and Aetiology of Congenitally Deafblind People in Denmark. *International Journal of Audiology, 49,* 76-82.

Dammeyer, J. (2010d). Interaction of Dual Sensory Loss, Cognitive Function and Communication in People Who are Congenitally Deaf-Blind. *Journal of Visual Impairment and Blindness, 104*(11), 719-725.

Dammeyer, J. (2011). Mental and Behavioral Disorders among People with Congenital Deaf Blindness. *Research in Developmental Disabilities, 32*(2), 571-575.

Dammeyer, J. (2012a). Children with Usher syndrome: mental and behavioral disorders. *Behavior and Brain Functions, 8*(16). doi:10.1186/1744-9081-8-16

Dammeyer, J. (2012b). Identification of Congenital Deaf-Blindness. *British Journal of Visual Impairment, 30*(2), 101-107.

Dekker, R., Drenth, P. J. D., Zaal, J. N., and Koole, F. D. (1990). An Intelligence Test Series for Blind and Low Vision Children. *Journal of Visual Impairment and Blindness, 84*, 71-76.

Duszak, R. S. (2009). Congenital Rubella Syndrome – Major Review. *Optometry, 80*, 36-43.

Edwards, L. and Crocker, S. (2008). *Psychological Processes in Deaf Children with Complex Needs. An Evidence-Based Practice Guide.* London: Jessica Kingsley Publishers.

Fellinger, J., Holzinger, D., and Polland, R. (2012). Mental Health of Deaf People. *The Lancet, 379,* 1037-1044.

Fellinger, J., Holzinger, D., Dirmhirn, A., van Dijk, J. and Goldberg, D. (2009). Failure to Detect Deaf-Blindness in a Population with Intellectual Disability. *Journal of Intellectual Disability Research, 53(10)*, 874-81.

Hallgren, B. (1959). Retinitis Pigmentosa Combined with Congenital Deafness; With Vestibulo-Cerebellar Ataxia and Mental Abnormality in a Proportion of Cases: A Clinical and Genetico-Statistical Study. *Acta Psychiatrica Scandinavica, 34*(Suppl.), 1-101.

Heiling, K. (1995). *The Development of Deaf Children: Academic Achievement Levels and Social Processes*. Hamburg, Germany: Signum.

Hendar, O. (2008). Goal fulfilment in school for the deaf and hearing impaired. Malmö, Sverige: Specialskolemyndigheten. Downloaded at: http://www.butiken.spsm.se/produkt/katalog_filer/2009_M%c3%a5luppfyllelse_ENG.pdf

Hendar, O. (2012). *Elever med Hörselshemming i Skolen – En Kartläggningsundersökelse om Läringsutbytte* [Pupils with hearing impairment and deafness – Education and outcome]. Oslo, Norge: Statped Skådalen (Utdanningsdirektoratet). Downloaded at: http://www.udir.no/Upload/Rapporter/2012/horsel.pdf?epslanguage=no

Hess-Röver, J., Crichton, J., Byrne, K. and Holland, A. J. (1999). Diagnosis and Treatment of a Severe Psychotic Illness in a Man with Dual Severe Sensory Impairments Caused by the Presence of Usher Syndrome. *Journal of Intellectual Disability Research, 43*(5), 428-434.

Hindley, P. (2000). Child and Adolescent Psychiatry. In Hindley, P. and Kitson, N. (Eds.): *Mental Health and Deafness*, pp. 42-74, London: Whurr.

Hindley, P. (2005). Mental health problems in deaf children. *Current Pediatrics*, *15*, 114–119.

Hindley, P., Hill, P. D., McGuigan, S., and Kitson, N. (1994). Psychiatric Disorder in Deaf and Hearing Impaired Children and Young People: A Prevalence Study. *Journal of Child Psychology and Psychiatry, 35*, 917–934.

Hobson, R. P. and Bishop, M. (2003). The Pathogenesis of Autism: Insights from Congenital Blindness. *Philosophical Transaction of the Royal Society B, 358*(1430), 335-344.

Hoevenaars-van den Boom, M. A. A., Antonissen, A. C., Knoors, H., and Vervloed, M. P. (2009). Differentiating Characteristics of Deaf-Blindness and Autism in People with Congenital Deaf-Blindness and Profound intellectual disability. *Journal of Intellectual Disability Research, 53*(6), *548-558.*

Huber, M. (2005). Health-Related Quality of Life of Austrian Children and Adolescents with Cochlear Implants. *International Journal of Pediatric Otorhinolaryngology, 69*, 1089–1101.

Janssen, M. and Rødbroe, I. (2007). *Communication and Congenital Deafblindness II: Contact and Social Interaction.* Aalborg, Denmark: Materialecentret.

Jumaian, A. and Fergusson, K. (2003). Psychosis in a Patient with Usher Syndrome: A Case Report. *Eastern Mediterranean Health Journal, 9*, 215-218.

Jure, R., Rapin, I., and Tuchman, R. F. (1991). Hearing-Impaired Autistic Children. *Developmental Medicine and Child Neurology, 33,* 1060-1072.

Karjalainen, S., Teräsvirta, M., Kärjä, J., and Kääriäinen, H. (1983). An Unusual Otological Manifestation of Usher's Syndrome in Four Siblings. *Clinical Genetics, 24*, 273-279.

Khan, S., Edwards, L., and Langdon, D. (2005). The Cognition and Behaviour of Children with Cochlear Implants, Children with Hearing Aids and their Hearing Peers: A comparison. *Audiology and Neuro-Otology, 10*(2), 117-126.

Klaver, C. C., Wolfs, R. C., Vingerling, J. R., Hofman, A., and de Jong, P. T. (1998). Age-specific Prevalence and Causes of Blindness and Visual Impairment in an Older Population. The Rotterdam Study. *Archives of Ophthalmology, 116*(5), 653-658.

Koizumi, J., Ofuku, K., Sakuma, K., Shiraishi, H., Iio, M., and Nawano, S. (1988). CNS changes in Usher's Syndrome with Mental Disorder: CT, MRI and PET Findings. *Journal of Neurology, Neurosurgery and Psychiatry, 51*(7), 987-990.

Korver, A. M. H., Admiraal, R. J. C., Kant, S. G., Dekker, F. W., Wever, C. C., Kunst, H. P. M., Frijns, J. H. M., and Oudesluys-Murphy, A. M. (2011). Causes of Permanent Childhood Hearing Impairment. *The Laryngoscope, 121*(2), 409-416.

Kvam, M. H., Loeb, M., and Tambs, K. (2006). Mental Health in Deaf Adults: Symptoms of Anxiety and Depression Among Hearing and Deaf Individuals. *Journal of Deaf Studies and Deaf Education, 12*(1), 1-7.

Ladd, P. (2003). *Understanding Deaf Culture. In Search of Deafhood.* Cleveton, UK: Multilingual Matters.

Laforge, R. G., Spector, W. D., and Sternberg, J. (1992). The Relationship Between Vision and Hearing Impairment to One-Year Mortality and Functional Decline. *Journal of Aging and Health, 4*(1), 126-148.

Lam. L. B., Christ, S. L., Lee, D. J., Zheng, D., and Arheart, K. L. (2008). Reported Visual Impairment and Risk of Suicide. The national 1986-1996 National Health Interview Surveys. *Archives of Ophthalmology, 126*(7), 975-980.

Lin, M. Y., Gutierrez, P. R., Stone, K. L., Yaffe, K., Ensrud, K. E., Fink, H. A., Sarkasian, C. A., Coleman, A. L. and Mangione, C. M. (2004). Vision Impairment and Combined Vision and Hearing Impairment Predict Cognitive and Functional Decline in Older Women. *Journal of the American Geriatrics Society, 52*(12), 1996-2002.

Lupsakko, T., Mantyjarvi, M., Kautiainen, H., and Sulkava, R. (2002). Combined hearing and visual impairment and depression in a population aged 75 years and older. *International Journal of Geriatric Psychiatry, 17*(9), *808-813.*

Maller, S. J. (1997). Deafness and WISC-III Item Difficulty: Invariance and Fit. *Journal of School Psychology, 35*(3), 299-314.

Mangotich, M. and Misiaszek, J. (1983). Atypical Psychosis in Usher's Syndrome. *Psychosomatics, 24*, 674-675.

Mayberry, R. I., (2003). Cognitive Development in Deaf Children: The Interface of Language and Perception in Neuropsychology. In Sagalowitz, S. J. and Rapin, I. (Eds.): *Handbook of Neuropsychology, Vol. 8, Part II,* 2nd ed., pp. 487-523. Amsterdam: Elsevier.

McDonald, C., Kenna, P., and Larkin, T. (1998). Retinitis Pigmentosa and Schizophrenia. *European Psychiatry, 13*, 423-426.

McDonnall, M. C. (2009). Risk Factors for Depression among Older Adults with Dual Sensory Loss. *Aging Mental Health, 13*(4), 569-576.

Meristo, M., Falkman, K., Hjelmquist, E., Tedoldi, M., Surian, L., and Siegal, M. (2007). Language Access and Theory of Mind Reasoning: Evidence from Deaf Children in Bilingual and Oral Environments. *Developmental Psychology, 43*(5), 1156-1169.

Mervis, C. A., Yeargin-Allsopp, M., Winter, S., and Boyle, C. (2000). Aetiology of Childhood Vision Impairment. Metropolitan Atlanta, 1991-93. *Paediatric and Perinatal Epidemiology, 14*(1), 70-77.

Meuwese-Jongejeugd, A., van Splunder, J., Vink, M., Stilma, J. S., van Zanten, B., Verschuure, H., Bernsen, R., and Evenhuis, H. (2008). Combined Sensory Impairment (Deaf-Blindness) in Five Percent of Adults with Intellectual Disabilities. *American Journal of Mental Retardation, 113*(4), 254-262.

Miner, I. D. (1995). Psychosocial Implications of Usher Syndrome, Type 1, Throughout the Life Cycle. *Journal of Visual Impairment and Blindness, 89*, 287-297.

Mukaddes, N. M., Lilincaslan, A., Kucukyazici, G., Sevketoglu, T., and Tuncer, S. (2007). Autism in Visually Impaired Individuals. *Psychiatry and Clinical Neuroscience, 61*(1), 39-44.

National Institute for Mental Health in England (2005). *Mental Health and Deafness – Towards Equity and Access*. London: Department of Health. Downloaded at: http://www.dh.gov.uk/prod_consum_dh/groups/dh_digitalassets/@dh/@en/documents/digitalasset dh_4104005.pdf

Nicholas, J. G. and Geers, A. E. (2003). Personal, Social and Family Adjustment in School-Aged Children with a Cochlear Implant. *Ear and Hearing, 24*(suppl.), 69–81.

Nuutila, A. (1970). Dystrophia Retinae Pigmentosa-Dysacusis Syndrome (DRD): A Study of the Usher- or Hallgren Syndrome. *Journal de Genetique Humaine, 18*, 57-88.

O'Donnell, N. (1991). *A Report on a Survey of Late Emerging Manifestations of Congenitally Rubella*. New York: Helen Keller National Center.

Owsley, C., McGwin, G. Jr., Scilley, K., Meek, G. C., Seker, D., and Dyer, A. (2007). Impact of Cataract Surgery on Health-Related Quality of Life in Nursing Home Residents. *British Journal of Ophthalmology, 91*, 1359–63.

Peterson, C. (2004). Theory of Mind Development in Oral Deaf Children with Cochlear Implants or Conventional Hearing Aids. *Journal of Child Psychology and Psychiatry, 45*(6), 1096-1106.

Peterson, C. and Siegal, M. (1999). Representing Inner Worlds: Theory of Mind in Autistic, Deaf and Normal Hearing Children. *Psychological Science, 10*(2), 126-129.

Polat, F. (2003). Factors Affecting Psychosocial Adjustment of Deaf Students. *Journal of Deaf Studies and Deaf Education, 8*, 325–339.

Preisler, G. (1991). Early Patterns of Interaction Between Blind Infants and Their Sighted Mothers. *Child: Care, Health and Development, 17*, 65-90.

Rais, T. (2006). Acute Psychosis with Paranoid Features in a Young Patient with Usher's Syndrome: A Case Report. *J Tenet Hum, 18*, 57-88.

Reagan, T G. (2010). *Language Policy and Planning for Sign Languages. Project MUSE.* Washington, DC: Gallaudet University Press.

Reinhardt, J. P. (1996). The Importance of Friendship and Family Support in Adaptation to Chronic Vision Impairment. *Journal of Gerontology: Psychology Science, 51B*(5), 268-278.

Rijavec, N. and Grubic, V. N. (2009). Usher Syndrome and Psychiatric Symptoms: A Challenge in Psychiatric Management. *Psychiatria Danubina, 21*, 68-71.

Roid, G. H. and Miller, L. J. (1997). *Examiner's Manual, Leiter International Performance Scale – Revised.* Wheat Lane, IL: Stoelting Company.

Ronnberg, J., and Borg, E. (2001). A Review and Evaluation of Research on the Deaf-Blind from Perceptual, Communicative, Social and Rehabilitative Perspectives. *Scandinavian Audiology, 30*(2), 67-77.

Schaefer, G. B., Bodensteiner, J. B., Thompson, J. N. Jr., Thompson, J. N. Jr., Kimberling, W. J., and Craft, J. M. (1998). Volumetric Neuroimaging in Usher Syndrome: Evidence of Global Involvement. *American Journal of Medical Genetics, 79*(1), 1-4.

Schneider, J., Gopinath, B., McMahon, C., Teber. E., Leeder, S. R., Wang, J. J., and Mitchell, P. (2012). Prevalence and 5-Year Incidence of Dual Sensory Impairment in an Older Australian Population. Annals of Epidemiology, 22(4)*, 295-301.*

Sever, J. L., South, M. A., and Shaver, K. A. (1985). Delayed Manifestations of Congenital Rubella. *Review of Infectious Diseases, 7*(S1), 164–169.

Sharp, C. W., Muir, W. J., Blackwood, D. H., Walker, M., Gosden, C., and St Clair, D. M. (1994). Schizophrenia and Mental Retardation Associated in a Pedigree with Retinitis Pigmentosa and Sensorineural Deafness. *American Journal of Medical Genetics, 54*, 354-360.

Sinkkonen, J. (1994). *Hearing Impairment, Communication and Personality Development.* Helsinki, Finland: Gummerus Kirjapaino Oy Jyväskylä.

Steinberg, A., Barnett, S., Meador, H. E., Wiggins, E., and Zazove, P. (2006). Health care system accessibility: experiences and perceptions of deaf people. *Journal of General Internal Medicine, 21*, 260-266.

Stevenson J., McCann D., Watkin P., Worsfold S., and Kennedy, C. (2010). The Relationship between Language Development and Behaviour Problems in Children with Hearing Loss. *Journal of Child Psychology and Psychiatry, 51*(1), 77-83.

Tambs, K. (2004). Moderate Effects of Hearing Loss on Mental Health and Subjective Well-Being: Results from the Nord-Trøndelag Hearing Loss Study. *Psychosomatic Medicine*, *66*, 776–782.

van Eyken, E., van Camp, G., and van Laer, L. (2007). The Complexity of Age-Related Hearing Impairment: Contributing Environmental and Genetic Factors. *Audiology and Neurotology, 12*(6), 345-358.

van Naarden, K., Decouflé, P., and Caldwell, K. (1999). Prevalence and Characteristics of Children with Serious Hearing Impairment. In Metropolitan Atlanta, 1991–1993. *Pediatrics, 103*, 570–575.

Viala, A., Nicot, T., Levy, F., and Vacheron, M. N. (2009). A case of Usher's Syndrome Associated with Psychotic Symptoms: Diagnosis and Follow-Up in a Psychiatric Unit. *Encephale, 35*, 286-291.

Warren, D. H. and Hatton, D. D. (2003). Cognitive Development in Children with Visual Impairments. In S. J. Segalowitz and I. Rapin (Eds): *Handbook of Neuropsychology*, 2nd Edition, Vol. 8, Part II. London: Elsevier.

Watkin, P. M. and Baldwin, M. (2011). Identifying Deafness in Early Childhood: Requirements after the Newborn Hearing Screen. *Archives of Diseases in Childhood, 96*, 62-66.

Waxham, M. N. and Wolinsky, J. S. (1984). Rubella Virus and its Effects on the Central Nervous System. *Neurological Clinics, 2*, 367-385.

Webster, W. S. (1998). Teratogen Update: Congenital Rubella. *Teratology, 58*, 13–23.

Werngren-Elgstrom, M., Dehlin, O., and Iwarsson, S. (2003). Aspects of Quality of Life in Persons with Prelingual Deafness Using Sign Language: Subjective Wellbeing, Ill-Health Symptoms, Depression and Insomnia. *Archives of Gerontology and Geriatrics, 37*, 13-24.

Wu, C. Y. and Chiu, C. C. (2006). Usher Syndrome with Psychotic Symptoms: Two Cases in the Same Family. *Psychiatry and Clinical Neuroscience, 60*, 626-628.

In: Mental Health and Psychiatry ISBN: 978-1-62417-589-3
Editors: A.S. Wilson and M.S. Schneider

Chapter 3

FURTHER EVIDENCE FOR EPIDEMIOLOGICAL TRANSITION HYPOTHESIS FOR ELDERLY SUICIDES

Ajit Shah[1,], Ravi Bhat[2] and Sofia Zarate-Escudero[3]*

[1]School of Health, University of Central Lancashire, Preston, United Kingdom

[2]Rural Health Academic Centre, University of Melbourne and Centre for Older Persons' Health, Shepparton, Victoria, Australia

[3]West London Mental Health NHS Trust, London, United Kingdom

ABSTRACT

Background: An epidemiological transition hypothesis has been theoretically developed and substantiated using one measure of socio-economic status (gross national domestic product [GDP]) to simultaneously explain wide cross-national variations in elderly suicide rates, trends over time for elderly suicide rates and age-associated trends

* Address for correspondence: 49 Erlesmere Gardens, Ealing, London W13 9TZ, United Kingdom. Telephone: 44 208 567 0829. Fax: 44 208 567 0829. E-mail: ajitshah123@btinternet.com.

in suicides rates. A curvilinear (inverted U-shaped curve) relationship between elderly suicide rates and GDP fitting the quadratic equation $Y = A + BX - CX^2$ (where Y is the suicide rate, X is the GDP and A,B, and C are constants) has been observed in a large cross-national study.

Methods: The predicted curvilinear relationship between elderly suicide rates and the Gini coefficient, another measure of socio-economic status (income inequality), fitting the above quadratic equation was examined with curve estimation regression model using data from the World Health Organisation.

Results: The relationship between suicide rates in both sexes in the age-bands 65-74 and 75+ years and the Gini coefficient was curvilinear and fitted the above quadratic equation, and was statistically significant (at least $P<0.05$) in all four groups.

Conclusions: Caution should be exercised in accepting this model of the epidemiological transition hypothesis for elderly suicide rates because it was generated from cross-sectional data using an ecological design. However, the previously observed relationship was replicated by using a different measure of socio-economic status. Ideally, this model requires rigorous testing by following selected low socio-economic status countries, over time, as they develop socio-economically.

INTRODUCTION

A developmental model of epidemiological transition for elderly suicide rates with four sequential stages was theoretically developed to simultaneously explain cross-national variations in elderly suicide rates, trends over time for elderly suicide rates and age-associated trends in suicides rates reported in the literature (Shah and Bhat, 2009).

This model was adapted from similar epidemiological transition models for dementia (Suh and Shah, 2001) and other mental disorders in old age (Shah, 2007). Although different countries will be at different stages of development within this model, it was proposed that each country would sequentially progress through the four stages over time with its socio-economic development.

Moreover, this model assumes that both socio-economic status and suicide rates can be dichotomised into two groups: high and low. The four sequential stages in this model were: low elderly suicide rate-low socio-economic society stage; high elderly suicide rate-low socio-economic society stage; high elderly suicide rate-high socio-economic society stage; and, low elderly suicide rate-high socio-economic society stage.

Low Elderly Suicide Rate-Low Socio-Economic Society Stage

Low socio-economic status was associated with low rates of suicide in the general population (Zhang, 1998; Simpson and Conklin, 1989) and in elderly men (Shah *et al.,* 2008a). Higher income inequality was also associated with lower suicide rates in the general population (Kowalski *et al.,* 1987; Vijaykumar *et al.,* 2005) and in the elderly (Shah *et al.,* 2008a; Redaniel *et al.,* 2011). Other markers of economic adversity, including higher housing loan interest rates, were associated with lower elderly suicide rates (Berk *et al.,* 2006). Societies with low socio-economic status have poorly developed healthcare services (Shah, 2007, 2009a; Jacob *et al.,* 2007; Jacob, 2008; Shah *et al.,* 2008a; Shah and Bhat, 2008a,b). Poorly developed healthcare services may mediate an increase in child mortality rates by being unable to provide primary preventative measures for diseases in childhood (e.g. immunisation programmes) and treatment for diseases that are directly related to low socio-economic status (e.g. infectious diseases) (Suh and Shah, 2001). Child mortality rates are higher in countries with low socio-economic status and higher income inequality (Zhang, 1998; Shah *et al*., 2008a; Shah, 2007). Increased child mortality rates will, in turn, reduce the life expectancy (Zhang, 1998; Shah *et al.,* 2008a; Shah, 2007). Given that suicide rates generally increase with age (Shah and De, 1998), reduced life expectancy will result in fewer people reaching the age of increased risk for suicide in societies with low socio-economic status. This, in turn, will result in a reduced number of elderly suicides in countries with low socio-economic status because there is a positive correlation between elderly suicide rates and elderly population size (Keimo, 2004; Shah *et al.,* 2008a) and elderly dependency ratios (Shah *et al.,* 2008b). Also, selective survival of those at reduced risk of suicide in old age due to genetic or constitutional factors may further compound this trend (Suh and Shah, 2001). Moreover, in societies with low socio-economic status, those who do survive into old age may be at reduced risk of suicide because they may be able to better tolerate additional hardship in old age due to life-long exposure to adversity (Lindesay, 1991; Seiden, 1981; McIntosh, 1984).

The above approach is consistent with a previously demonstrated model with five sequential stages (Shah *et al*., 2008a): (i) presence of a low socio-economic status; (ii) low socio-economic status leading to poorly developed healthcare services; (iii) poorly developed healthcare services may interact, mediate and modify other factors and contribute to increased child mortality rates; (iv) increased child mortality rates leading to reduced life expectancy; and, (v) reduced life expectancy leading to fewer people reaching the age of increased risk of suicide, and resulting in low elderly suicide rates in societies with low socio-economic status. This situation could be labelled as a low elderly suicide rate-low socio-economic society stage.

High Elderly Suicide Rate-Low Socio-Economic Society Stage

With improvement in the socio-economic status of countries, the degree of development of healthcare services will also improve (Zhang, 1998; Shah, 2007, 2009a; Jacob *et al.,* 2007; Shah *et al.,* 2008a; Shah and Bhat, 2008). Improvement in healthcare services may facilitate reduction in child mortality rates because of improved ability to provide primary preventative measures for diseases in childhood (e.g. immunisation programmes) and treatment for diseases that are directly related to low socio-economic status (e.g. infectious diseases) (Suh and Shah, 2001). Reduction in child mortality rates will, in turn, increase the life expectancy (Zhang, 1998; Keimo, 2005; Shah, 2007; Shah *et al.,* 2008a). This, in turn, will result in greater number of subjects reaching the age of increased risk of suicide and an increase in elderly suicide rates (Shah *et al.,* 2008a). This approach is also consistent with the five stage sequential model described above in the section on Low elderly suicide rates – low socio-economic society stage (Shah *et al.,* 2008a). This will lead to a gradual transition from low elderly suicide rate-low socio-economic society stage to a high elderly suicide rate-low socio-economic society stage.

High Elderly Suicide Rate-High Socio-Economic Society Stage

As societies develop they are likely to change from being socio-economically less developed to being socio-economically more developed (Zhang, 1998; Shah, 2007, 2009a; Jacob *et al.,* 2007; Shah and Bhat, 2008a,b; Shah *et al.,* 2008a). Further improvement in healthcare services may facilitate further reductions in child mortality rates because of improved ability to provide primary preventative measures for diseases in childhood (e.g. immunisation programmes) and treatment for diseases that are directly related to low socio-economic status (e.g. infectious diseases) (Suh and Shah, 2001). Further reductions in child mortality rates will, in turn, further increase the life expectancy (Zhang, 1998; Keimo, 2004; Shah, 2007; Shah *et al.,* 2008a). This, in turn, will result in increasing number of subjects reaching the age of increased risk of suicide (Shah *et al.,* 2008a). Reduced child mortality rates and increased life expectancy will also lead to reduction in selective survival of those at reduced risk of suicide in old age due to constitutional or genetic factors.

Furthermore, the protective effects of life-long adversity on elderly suicide rates (McIntosh, 1984; Seiden, 1981; Lindesay, 1991) may be absent in countries with higher socio-economic status. Another factor is the influence of poor availability and/or access to appropriate care in people from socio-economically deprived communities in countries with high socio-economic status (Kivimäki *et al.,* 2007), and the elderly are particularly likely to be socio-economically deprived. The composite effect of these changes would be an increase in the number of individuals at increased risk of suicide in old age in socio-economically more developed societies. This approach is also consistent with the five stage sequential model described above in the section on Low elderly suicide rates – low socio-economic society stage (Shah *et al.,* 2008a). This will lead to a gradual transition from the high elderly suicide rate-low socio-economic society stage to a high elderly suicide rate-high socio-economic society stage.

Low Elderly Suicide Rate-High Socio-Economic Society Stage

Theoretically, in socio-economically well developed societies, due to further reduction in child mortality rates and increase in life expectancy, greater number of people would reach the age of increased of suicide, and consequently lead to higher elderly suicide rates. However, in many socio-economically well developed countries (e.g. Italy, Netherlands, Norway, United Kingdom and United States) elderly suicide rates were comparatively low (Shah *et al.,* 2007) and declined over time (Shah *et al.,* 2008c). The five stage sequential model described above in the section on Low elderly suicide rates – low socio-economic status society stage (Shah *et al.*, 2008a) may not apply to socio-economically very well developed societies. In socio-economically very well developed societies, elderly suicide rates may progressively decline over many years due to improved efforts to control the risk factors for elderly suicides, enhance protective factors for elderly suicides, advances in medical care, prompt resuscitation of those who attmept suicide, better provision of healthcare (including mental health) services and public health initiatives to reduce suicide rates (Gunnell *et al.,* 2003; Kua *et al.,* 2003; Lodhi and Shah, 2004, 2005; Yip et al., 2005; Shah and Coupe, 2009; Shah, 2009b). Ultimately, this will lead to a gradual transition from a high elderly suicide rate-high socio-economic society stage to a low elderly suicide rate-high socio-economic society stage.

The epidemiological transition model proposed above would follow an inverted U-shaped curve with a quadratic pattern ($Y= A + BX - CX^2$, where A, B and C are constants, Y is the elderly suicide rates and X is the measure of socio-economic status). The relationship between suicide rates in both sexes in the age-bands 65-74 and 75+ years and the gross national domestic product (GDP) was observed to be curvilinear (inverted U-shaped curve) fitting the above quadratic equation, and was statistically significant (at least at $P<0.05$) in all four groups, in a recent cross-national study of 105 countries (Shah, 2010). This provided support for the epidemiological transition hypothesis for elderly suicide rates. However, caution should be exercised in accepting this model because it was generated from cross-sectional data using an ecological design. With this in view, this current study aims to replicate the findings using a different measure of socio-economic status, the Gini coefficient (a measure of income inequality and inversely correlated with the GDP) (Shah, 2007).

METHODS

Suicide Rates

Data on suicide rates for males and females in the age-bands 65-74 and 75+ years was ascertained from the WHO (http://www.who.int/whosis/database/mort/table1.cfm).

For a small number of countries only the raw figures for the number of suicides were available from the WHO website. Suicide rates for such countries were calculated by dividing the number of reported suicides by the population size in the relevant age-band and sex group available on the same website. Data were ascertained for the latest year.

Data on Socio-Economic Status and Other Variables

The Gini coefficient has been used as a measure for socio-economic status of countries in previous studies of suicide rates (Shah *et al.,* 2008a). The Gini coefficient is derived from an income distribution curve where the x-axis represents the number of households and the y-axis percentage of the total income. Perfect equality is seen when the income is equally distributed across all the households and perfect inequality is seen when only one household has all the income.

The area between the line of perfect equality and the actual income distribution is the Gini coefficient and is expressed as a percentage ranging form 0 (perfect equality) to 100% (perfect inequality). The United Nations Development Programme website (www.hdr.undp.org/reports/global/ 2005/ pdf/hdr05_HDI.pdf) provided data on the Gini coefficient.

Data on per capita expenditure on healthcare, the proportion of Gross National Domestic Product (GDP) spent on healthcare and child mortality rates have collectively been used as proxy measures of the quality and quantity of healthcare services (Shah, 2007; Shah *et al.,* 2008a). Data on per capita expenditure on healthcare and the proportion of GDP spent on healthcare, life expectancy and child mortality rates were ascertained from the WHO website (http://www.who.int/countries/afg/en/) for the year 2006.

Data Analysis

The relationship between suicide rates and the Gini coefficient was examined with curve estimation regression model in order to test the "a priori" hypothesis of a curvilinear relationship (inverted U-shaped curve) fitting the quadratic equation $Y = A + BX - CX^2$ (where Y is the suicide rate, X is the Gini coefficient, and A,B, and C are constants).

The relationships between suicide rates and per capita expenditure on healthcare, the proportion of GDP spent on healthcare, life expectancy and child mortality rates were examined with Spearman's correlation coefficient. The inter-relationships between the Gini coefficient and per capita expenditure on healthcare, the proportion of GDP spent on healthcare, life expectancy and child mortality rates were also examined with Spearman's correlation coefficient.

Sensitivity of the Data Analysis

The median for the year of the suicide rate data was 2005, but the range was very wide (1970-2007); the median for the year for Gini coefficient data was 2000, but the range was very wide (1992-2003). Therefore, the curvilinear relationship between elderly suicide rates and the Gini coefficient was reexamined with curve estimation regression model for countries with recent data (for the year 2000 or more recent) for elderly suicide rates and the Gini coefficient.

Additional sensitivity analysis were conducted by using the average suicide rates calculated from the available suicide rates for the latest five years for both sexes in both the elderly age-bands.

RESULTS

Data on both elderly suicide rates and the Gini coefficient were available for 80 countries. The median (range) for the year of the suicide rate data was 2005 (1970-2007). The median (range) for the year for Gini coefficient data was 2000 (1992-2003). Table 1 describes the descriptive characteristics of the elderly suicide rates in both sexes in both the elderly age-bands and the Gini coefficient.

Curve Regression Analyses

Table 2 illustrates the characteristics of the curve estimation regression models for males and females in both the elderly age-bands. The relationship between suicide rates in males and females in the age-bands 65-74 years and 75+ years and the Gini coefficient was curvilinear (inverted U-shaped curve) and fitted the quadratic equation $Y = A + BX - CX^2$; this relationship was statistically significant (at least $P<0.05$) in all four groups.

Table 1. Basic characteristics of suicide rates and GDP

	Median	Range
* *Suicide Rates*:		
Males Aged 65-74 years	17.1	0-95.90
Males aged 75+ years	29.2	0-154.8
Females aged 65-74 years	5.1	0-39.2
Females aged 75+ years	5.75	0-70.30
Gini coefficient	36.0	1.9-59.2

* Suicide rates were per 100,000 of the relevant age and sex groups in the general population.

Table 2. Curve estimation regression models for the relationship between elderly suicide rates and the GDP

	R^2	Degrees of Freedom	F Value	Significance	Regression Equation
Curve estimation regression:					
Males 65-74 years	0.13	77	5.48	P=0.006	$Y = 24.83 + 0.75X - 0.018X^2$
Males 75+ years	0.15	77	6.62	P=0.002	$Y = 41.38 + 0.99X - 0.027X^2$
Females 65-74 years	0.15	77	6.67	P=0.002	$Y = 12.69 - 0.010X - 0.003X^2$
Females 75+ years	0.11	77	4.7	P=0.011	$Y = 4.22 + 0.68X - 0.013X^2$

Y = Suicide rates.
X = Gini coefficient.
A, B and C are constants.

Sensitivity Analyses

The findings from the sensitive analysis, by only including the 51 countries with recent data (for the year 2000 or more recent) on suicide rates and the Gini coefficient, were similar for the curve regression analyis. The findings from the sensitivity analysis using the average suicide rates calculated from the latest five years data on suicide rates, from 73 countries, were similar for the curve regression analysis.

Other Correlations

Table 3 illustrates the correlations between elderly suicide rates and per capita expenditure on healthcare, the proportion of the GDP spent on healthcare, life expectancy and child mortality rates. There were significant positive correlations between suicide rates in both sexes in both the elderly age-bands and per capita expenditure on healthcare. There was a significant positive correlations between suicide rates in males and females in both elderly age-bands and the per capita healthcare expenditure; there was a postive correlation between suicide rates in males aged 75+ years and the proportion of GDP spent on healthcare.

Table 3. The relationship between elderly suicide rates and other measured variables

Suicide Rates(N=79)	Per Capita Healthcare Expenditure	Proportion GDP spent on Healthcare	Life Expectancy Males	Life Expectancy Females	Child Mortality Males	Child Mortality Females
Males 65-74 years	Rho=+0.40 P<0.0001	NS	Rho=+0.21 P=0.06		Rho=-0.53 P<0.0001	
Males 75+ years	Rho=+0.49 P<0.0001	Rho=+0.27 P=0.015	Rho=+0.27 P=0.015		Rho=-0.56 P<0.0001	
Females 65-74 years	Rho=+0.43 P<0001	NS		Rho=+0.39 P<0001		Rho=-0.55 P<0.0001
Females 75+ years	Rho=+0.39 P<0.0001	NS		Rho=+0.32 P=0.004		Rho=-0.49 P<0.0001

NS=Not significant.

There were significant positive correlations between suicide rates in males aged 75+ years and females aged 65-74 years and 75+ years and life expectancy (the correlation with males aged 65-74 years approached significance). There were significant negative correlations between suicide rates in both sexes in both the elderly age-bands and child mortality rates.

The Gini coefficient was significantly negatively correlated with per capita expenditure on healthcare (Rho=-0.37, P=0.001) and female life expectancy (Rho=-0.30, P=0.008), and significantly positively correlated with male (Rho=+0.45, P<0.00001) and female (Rho=+0.47, P<0.00001) child mortality rates; the relationship with male expectancy approached significance (Rho=-0.2, P=0.086). The per capita expenditure on healthcare was significantly positively correlated with the proportion of GDP spent on healthcare (Rho=+0.63, P<0.00001), life expectancy for males (Rho=+0.79, P<0.00001) and females (Rho=+0.87, P<0.00001), and significantly negatively correlated with male (Rho=-0.85, P<0.00001) and female (Rho=-0.84, P<0.00001) child mortality rates. The proportion of GDP spent on healthcare was significantly positively correlated with life expectancy for males (Rho=+0.48, P<0.0001) and females (Rho=+0.50, P<0.0001) and significantly negatively correlated with male (Rho=-0.41, P<0.0001) and female (Rho=-0.40, P<0.0001) child mortality rates. There was a significant negative correlation between life expectancy and child mortality rates for males (Rho=-0.79, P<0.00001) and females (Rho=-0.90, P<0.0001).

Discussion

Some methodological issues need consideration. Cross-national data on suicide rates should be viewed cautiously because: data were not available from all countries (Moscicki, 1995; Wasserman *et al.,* 2005); the validity of this data was unclear (Diekstra, 1989; Wasserman *et al.,* 2005); the legal criteria for the proof of suicide vary between countries and in different regions within a country (Shah and Ganesvaran, 1994; Wasserman *et al*., 2005); some countries, particularly low-income countries, may have poor death registration facilities (Shah and Ganesvaran, 1994); and, cultural and religious factors and stigma attached to suicide may lead to under-reporting of suicides (Wasserman *et al.,* 2005; Abraham *et al.,* 2005). Data on socio-economic status and health-related measures should also be viewed with caution because: the validity of this data is unclear; some countries may have poor registration facilities for data on health-related measures; some countries may have poor infrastructure for providing accurate financial data (Shah *et al.,* 2008a); and, their influence on social distribution of risk factors may be complex (Lynch *et al.,* 2004). These latter concerns are more likely to be observed in low-income countries. Also, the influence of other variables was not controlled for in the curve regression analysis because this is not possible with curve regression models where only the relationship between two variables can be examined. GDP is an important variable in this context because socio-economic status the Gini coefficient and the GDP are inversely correlated (Shah *et al.,* 2008a), but it was not possible to control for this variable. However, data were gathered from the WHO and United Nations Website data banks and were the latest and best available data set. Moreover, in the sensitivity analysis the findings of the curve estimation regression models were similar for the entire data set and for countries with more recent data (for the year 2000 or more recent) on suicide rates and the Gini coefficient, and when the average suicide rates of the suicide rates for the latest five years were used. Furthermore, similar findings have been published for the relationship between elderly suicides rates and urbanization using WHO data on suicide rates for different years supporting the validity of using WHO suicide rate data in ecological studies (Shah, 2009c). Also, the relationship between elderly suicide rates and data on psychiatric funding, policy and service provision from two sources several years apart were identical again supporting the validity of using WHO suicide rate data in ecological studies (Shah and Bhat, 2008a)..

The findings of significant curvilinear (inverted U-shaped curve) relationships between suicide rates in both sexes in both the elderly age-bands and the Gini coefficient fitting the quadratic equation $Y = A + BX - CX^2$ confirmed the "a priori" study hypothesis. Moreover, the findings confirmed previously observed identical relationship between elderly suicide rates and another measure of socio-economic status (GDP) (Shah, 2010). This may be an artefact of the methodological issues described. However, there is supporting evidence, consistent with the literature, suggesting that the finding may be genuine and is examined below.

The inter-correlations between per capita expenditure on healthcare, the proportion of GDP spent on health, life expectancy and child mortality rates, and between these variables and both elderly suicide rates and the Gini coefficient were consistent with the literature and supported the theoretical background used in developing the epidemiological transition hypothesis – both described in detail in the Introduction. First, the negative correlations between the Gini coefficient and per capita expenditure on healthcare suggests that health care services may be poorly developed in countries with low socio-economic status, and is consistent with the literature (Shah, 2007, 2009a; Jacob *et al.,* 2007; Shah *et al.,* 2008a; Shah and Bhat, 2008a,b). Second, both per capita expenditure on healthcare and the proportion of GDP spent on healthcare were significantly and negatively correlated with child mortality rates, and is consistent with the literature (Zhang, 1998; Shah *et al.*, 2008a; Shah, 2007). Poorly developed healthcare services may mediate an increase in child mortality rates by being unable to provide primary preventative measures for diseases in childhood (e.g immunisation programmes) and treatment for diseases that are directly related to low socio-economic status (e.g infectious diseases) (Suh and Shah, 2001). Third, child mortality rates were significantly and negatively correlated with life expectancy, and this is consistent with the literature (Zhang, 1998; Shah *et al.,* 2008a; Shah, 2007). This observation also supports each of the four stages of the epidemiological transition hypothesis of elderly suicide rates. Given that suicide rates generally increase with age (Shah and De, 1998), reduced life expectancy will result in fewer people reaching the age of increased risk for suicide in societies with low socio-economic status. Finally, there were generally significant and positive correlations between life expectancy and elderly suicide rates and is also consistent with the literature (Shah *et al.,* 2008a). Collectively, these observations support each of the first three stages of the epidemiological transition hypothesis of elderly suicide rates and they also partly support the fourth stage. Furthermore, the generally significant correlations between elderly suicide rates and per capita expenditure on healthcare (positive), the proportion of GDP spent on health (positive), child mortality rates (negative) and life expectancy (positive) also support each of the first three stages of the epidemiological transition hypothesis of elderly suicide rates and they also partly support the fourth stage. This study, using a different measure of socio-economic status (Gini coefficient), has replicated the earlier finding of a curvelinear relationship between elderly suicide rates and GDP and suggests that this finding is robust. However, caution should be exercised in accepting this model of the epidemiological transition hypothesis for elderly suicide rates because it has been generated from cross-sectional data using an ecological design and is subject to ecological fallacy. It is, therefore, difficult to be conclusive about the aetiological implications and the findings may merely be an association. Moreover, the variance in suicide rates explained by this inverted U-shaped curvilear relationship is small and thus other additional explanatory models also require investigation. Furthermore, the influence of socio-economic status on elderly suicide rates may interact with, mediate or modify the effect of other factors not examined in this study. These factors include cross-national differences in rural/urban location, the distribution of protective and risk factors, in the prevalence of mental illness in different age and sex groups (Shah *et al.*, 2007), genetic factors that differentially predispose different age and sex groups to mental illness or directly to suicidal behaviour (Shah *et al.*,, 2007), cultural factors with differential influence on different age and sex groups (Yip et al., 2005; Kua et al., 2003), and cohort effects with differential influence on different age and sex groups (Woodbury et al., 1987; Gunnell et al., 2004). Ideally, this model requires rigorous testing by following selected low socio-economic status countries, over time, as they develop socio-economically; if this model is accurate then such countries would go through all four stages and the changes would follow the predicted curvilinear (inverted U-shaped) relationship.

Declaration of Interests

None

Role of Authors

AS and RB conceived the idea for this study based on their collaboration on many suicide studies. AS collected the suicide data and RB provided the

Gini coefficient data. AS conducted the data analysis and wrote the first draft. All authors improved the first draft. RB and SZ conducted an updated literature search. SZ is a trainee learning research methodology.

References

Abrahams, V.J., Abrahams, S and Jacob, K.S. (2005). Suicide in the elderly in Kanyambadi block, Tamil Nadu, South India. *International Journal of Geriatric Psychiatry*, 20, 953-955.

Berk, M., Dodd, S and Henry, M. (2006). The effect of macroeconomic variables on suicide. *Psychological Medicine*, 36, 181-189.

Diekstra, R.F.W. (1989). Suicide and attemptede suicide: an international perspective. *Acta Psychiatrica Scandinavica*, 80 (Suppl 354), 1-24.

Gunnell, D., Middleston, N., Whitley, E., Dorling, D and Frankel, S. (2003). Why are suicide rates rising in young men but falling in the elderly? – a time-series analysis of trends in England and Wales 1950-1998. *Social Science and Medicine*, 57, 595-611.

Gunnell, D., Middleston, N., Whitley, E., Dorling, D and Frankel, S. (2004). Influence of cohort effects on paterrns of suicide in England and Wales, 1950-1999. *British Journal of Psychiatry*, 182, 164-170.

Jacob, K.S. (2008). The prevention of suicide in India and the developing world: the need for population-based strategies. *Crisis,* 29(2): 102-6.

Jacob, K.S., Sharan, P., Mirza, I., Garrido-Cumbrera, M., Seedat, S., Mari, J.J. and Sreen, V. (2007). Global mental health 4. Mental health systems in countries: where are we now?. *Lancet*, 370, 1061-1077.

Kiemo, K. (2004). Towards a socio-economic and demographic theory of elderly suicides: a comparison of 49 countries at various stages of development. www.soc.ou.se/publications/fulltext/diss2003-3.pdf. Viewed 2 Febraury 2007.

Kivimäki, M., Gunnell, D., Lawlor, D.A., Davey Smith, G., Pentti, J., Virtanen, M., Elovainio, M., Klaukka, T. and Vahtera, J. (2007). Social inequalities in antidepressant treatment and mortality: a longitudinal register study. *Psychological Medicine*, 37 (3): 373-82.

Kowalski, G.S., Faupel, C.E and Starr, P.D. (1987). Urbanisation and suicides: a study of American Counties. *Social Forces*, 66, 85-101.

Kua, E.H., Ko, S.M and Ng, T.P. (2003). Recent trends in elderly suicide rates in a multi-ethnic Asian city. *International Journal of Geriatric Psychiatry*, 18, 533-536.

Lindesay, J. (1991). Suicide in the elderly. *International Journal of Geriatric Psychiatry*, 6, 355-361.

Lodhi, L and Shah, A.K. (2004). Psychotropic prescriptions and elderly suicide rates. *Medicine, Science and the Law*, 44, 236-244.

Lodhi, L and Shah, A.K. (2005). Factors associated with the recent decline in suicide rates in England and Wales. 1985-1998. *Medicne, Science and the Law*, 45, 115-120.

Lynch, J., Davey Smith, G, Harpe, S. et al (2004). Is income inequality a determinant of population health? Part 1. A systematic review. *Millbank Q*, 82, 5-99.

McIntosh, J.L. (1984). Components of the decline in elderly suicides: suicide in young old and old old by race and sex. *Death Education*, 8, 113-124.

Moscicki, E.K. (1995). North American perspectives: epidemiology of suicide. *International Psychogeriatrics*, 7, 137-148.

Redaniel, M.T., Lebanan-Dalida, M.A. and Gunnell, D. (2011). Suicide in the Philippines: time trend analysis (1974-2005) and literature review. *BMC Public Health*, 6 (11): 536.

Seiden, R.H. (1981). Mellowing with age: factors affecting the non-white suicide rate. *International Journal of Ageing and Human Development*, 13, 265-284.

Shah, A.K and Bhat, R. (2008a). The relationship between elderly suicide rates and mental health funding, service provision and national policy: a cross-national study. *International Psychogeriatrics*, 20, 605-615.

Shah, A.K and Bhat, R. (2008b). Are elderly suicide rates improved by increased provision of mental health service resources? *International Psychogeriatrics*, 20, 1230-1237.

Shah, A.K and Bhat, R. (2009). Development of an Epidemiological transition model to explain cross-national variations in elderly suicide rates, time trends in elderly suicide rates and age-associated trends in suicide rates. *Psychiatric Research Journal*, 1 (3): 241-256.

Shah, A.K and Coupe, J. (2009). A comparative study of elderly suicides in England and Wales, Scotland and Northern Ireland: trends over time and age-associated trends. *International Psychogeriatrics*. In Press.

Shah, A.K and De, T. (1998). Suicide and the elderly. *International Journal of Psychiatry in Clinical Practice*, 2, 3-17.

Shah, A.K and Ganesvaran, T. (1994). Suicide in the elderly. *In: Functional Psychiatric Disorders of the Elderly (Eds. Chiu E, Ames D)*. Cambridge, Cambridge University Press. Pgs 221-244.

Shah, A.K. (2007). The importance of socio-economic status of countries for mental disorders in old age: a development of an epidemiological transition model. *International Psychogeriatrics*, 19, 785-787.

Shah, A.K. (2009a). The relationship between socio-economic status and mental health funding, service provision and national policy: a cross-national study. *International Psychiatry*, 6, 44-46.

Shah, A.K. (2009b). Attempted suicide in the elderly in England: age-associated rates, time trends and methods. *International Psychogeriatrics*. In Press.

Shah, A.K. (2009c). A Replication of Cross-National Study of the relationship between elderly Suicide Rates and Urbanisation. *International Psychogeriatrics*. In Press.

Shah, A.K. (2010). The possible evidence for epidemiological transition hypothesis for elderly suicides. *International Psychogeriatrics*, 22, 219-226.

Shah, A.K., Bhat, R., MacKenzie, S. and Koen, C. (2007). Elderly suicide rates: cross-national comparisons and association with sex and elderly age-bands. *Medicine, Science and the Law*, 47, 56-60.

Shah, A.K., Bhat, R., MacKenzie, S. and Koen, C. (2008a). A cross-national study of the relationship between elderly suicide rates and life expectancy and markers of socio-economic status and healthcare status. *International Psychogeriatrics*, 20, 347-360.

Shah, A.K., Bhat, R., MacKenzie, S. and Koen, C. (2008c). Elderly suicide rates: cross-national comparisons of trends over a 10-year period. *International Psychogeriatrics,* 20, 673-686.

Shah, A.K., Padayatchi, M. and Das, K. (2008b).The relationship between elderly suicide rates and elderly dependency ratios: a cross-national study using data from the WHO data bank. *International Psychogeriatrics*, 20, 594-604.

Simpson, M.E., Conklin, G.H. (1989). Socioeconomic development, suicide and religion: a test of Durkhiem's theory of religion and suicide. *Social Forces*, 67, 945-964.

Suh, G.H and Shah, A.K. (2001). A review of the epidemiological transition in dementia – cross-national comparisons of the indices related to Alzheimer's disease and vascular dementia. *Acta Psychiatrica Scandinavica*, 104, 4-11.

Vijayakumar, L., Nagaraj, K., Pirkis, J and Whiteford, H. (2005). Suicide in developing countries (1): frequency, distribution, and association with socio-economic indicators. *Crisis,* 26, 104-111.

Wasserman, D., Cheng, Q and Jiang, G.X. (2005). Global suicide rates among young people aged 15-19. *World Psychiatry*, 4, 114-120.

Woodbury, M.A., Manton, K.G and Blazer, D. (1987). Trends in US suicide mortality rates 1968-1982: race and sex differences in age, period and cohort components. *International Journal of Epidemiology*, 17, 356-352.

Yip, P.S.F., Liu, K.Y., Hu, J and Song, X.M. (2005). Suicide rates in China during a decade of rapid social change. *Social Psychiatry and Psychiatric Epidemiology*, 40, 792-798.

Zhang, J. (1998). Suicide in the world: toward a population increase theory of suicide. *Death Studies*, 22, 525-539.

In: Mental Health and Psychiatry ISBN: 978-1-62417-589-3
Editors: A.S. Wilson and M.S. Schneider

Chapter 4

THE PSYCHIATRY OF PELLAGRA: A FORGOTTEN DISEASE?

***Andrea E. Cavanna*[1,2*], *James W. Mitchell*[1] *and Adrian C. Williams*[3]**

[1]Department of Neuropsychiatry,
BSMHFT and University of Birmingham, United Kingdom
[2]Sobell Department of Motor Neuroscience and Movement Disorders,
UCL and Institute of Neurology, London, United Kingdom
[3]Department of Neurology, UHB and University of Birmingham,
United Kingdom

ABSTRACT

Pellagra is a systemic disease resulting from decreased cellular niacin and clinically presenting with the diagnostic triad of dermatitis, diarrhoea and dementia ('three Ds'). Although infrequently described in the pellagra literature, a number of neuropsychiatric symptoms other than dementia may present at any stage of the disease and affect a large proportion of patients. These include anxiety, depression and mania, as well as hallucinations, disturbances of thought and delusional beliefs. A number of personality changes have also been reported, resulting in social

* Correspondence: Prof Andrea E. Cavanna, MD, PhD, Department of Neuropsychiatry, The Barberry National Centre for Mental Health, Birmingham B152FG, United Kingdom, Email: A.Cavanna@ion.ucl.ac.uk.

isolation, violence and aggression. Finally, *ante litteram* Parkinsonian features have been identified since the earliest description of pellagra. In addition to the neuropsychiatric symptoms that may result from the disease, it should also be noted that certain psychiatric conditions, such as anorexia nervosa and alcohol dependence, may be the underlying reason for the dietary deficiency. Cases of pellagra are not rare in developing countries and may be on the increase in the developed world. It is important to consider the full neuropsychiatric spectrum of pellagra, particularly since a number of patients may present with a clinical picture which does not exactly match the 'classical' diagnostic triad (e.g. *pellagra sine pellagra*).

Keywords: Pellagra; Behaviour; Psychiatry; Anxiety; Depression; Psychosis; Dementia

INTRODUCTION

Pellagra is a systemic disease resulting from decreased cellular niacin, clinically presenting with the diagnostic triad of dermatitis, diarrhoea and dementia ('three Ds'). This can lead to death if treatment is not received. The disease is most commonly caused by dietary deficiency of the B vitamin niacin or its precursor tryptophan. Pellagra was first described in the mid-17th century by the Spanish physician Casal and was later given the name pellagra due to its dermatological manifestations (*pelle agra* meaning *rough/sour skin* in Italian) [1]. It became endemic in the poor regions of southern Europe, particularly in northern Italy throughout the 18th and 19th centuries [2]. In the early 20th century pellagra was highly prevalent the southern states of America, where it was the 8th or 9th most common cause for death by the end of the 1920s [3]. These states experienced a high level of poverty, with maize (a poor nutritional source of tryptophan and niacin) being the major food source for a large proportion of the population. Due to the fact that the disease was most prevalent where maize was the main food source, it was believed that the condition was due to an infectious agent or toxin within the maize [4] However, in 1914 Goldberger suggested that the disease was not infectious, but instead caused by dietary deficiency [5]. One of the reasons prompting the hypothesis, now known to be correct, was the low prevalence of the disease in hospital staff treating patients with pellagra. This claim was supported in his later studies which demonstrated that patients could recover from the disease by altering their diet to include fresh animal products and vegetables [6]. In later work, Goldberger demonstrated that the condition could be prevented by vitamin B in animal models [7], but it was not until after his death that niacin was found to be the curative agent in question [8] After this discovery, the United States introduced policy for widespread vitamin fortification of flour along with public awareness campaigns in an attempt to diversify the population's diet [9]. The consequence was almost complete eradication of the disease by the mid-20th century [10]. Although less common than at the start of the 20th century, pellagra still remains a problem in areas of humanitarian crisis. For example, the disease has recently been observed in more than 1 in 50 Mozambican refugees to Malawi as well as in refugee populations in Angola, Nepal and Zimbabwee.[11] In developed countries, the condition has been reported in homeless people with nutritionally unbalanced diets [12]. It is also reported in the context of anorexia nervosa and alcohol dependence, where there can be insufficient dietary intake of either niacin or tryptophan [13 14]. It should also be noted that the disease can present even if there is no dietary deficiency of the B vitamin. In the context of HIV infection the dermatitis, diarrhoea (AIDS enteropathy) and the AIDS dementia complex (ADC) may be explained by a virus-induced pellagra, evidenced by the concomitant serum tryptophan depletion in this population [15]. A pellagra-like syndrome is also described in patients with carcinoid syndrome, where tryptophan metabolism is shunted away from niacin production and towards serotonin (5-HT) synthesis [16]. This is also observed in patients receiving medications which affect niacin associated metabolic pathways, such isoniazid and 5-flurouracil [17 18].

Due to pellagra being a vitamin deficiency disease, there are a wide range of clinical characteristics which can present. Furthermore the clinical picture can vary widely from one patient to another, with some patients presenting with the classical diagnostic triad and others exhibiting less well defined symptoms. The hallmark sign in patients with pellagra is a symmetric erythematous rash which appears in sun-exposed areas. This tends to be on the dorsal aspect of the hands and forearms, the face and the upper part of the chest which is not shaded by the chin (leading to the characteristic 'Casals necklace' appearance). Vesicles and bullae may develop which may later rupture and the skin may become thick and hyperpigmented as the disease progresses. Patients also present with a number of gastrointestinal symptoms, the most well known being diarrhoea. Glossitis may also be observed and lead to mouth soreness and dysphagia and patients may experience nausea, vomiting and loss of appetite. The reduced oral intake of food and malabsoption which results from these symptoms can compound the niacin deficiency further [19]. The most widely known neurological manifestation of the disease is the dementia, although this characterisation may be misleading since the symptoms are generally more in line with delirium. In later stages, sensorimotor neuropathies and Parkinsonism may also be found [20]. In addition to the clinical manifestations defined above, pellagra is generally diagnosed if the patient gives a history of poor dietary intake of niacin and has decreased levels of urinary niacin metabolites. It should be noted, however, that many patients may present with a clinical picture which does not exactly match the 'classical' diagnostic triad (*pellagra sine pellagra*). Treatment by oral administration of nicotinamide is very successful [19]. Despite the well reported '3rd D' of the triad, dementia, there are a plethora of neuropsychiatric symptoms which can present throughout the disease process which are less well characterised. This chapter will focus on the neuropsychiatric aspects of the condition, using the current literature and reassessing the landmark pellagra studies, particularly from the United States in the early 20th century.

PATHOPHYSIOLOGY

Pellagra affects a number of organ systems due to the role that niacin plays in the synthesis of the important metabolic co-enzymes, nicotinamide adenine dinucleotide (NAD) and nicotinamide adenine dinucleotide phosphate (NADP). Both of these co-enzymes are involved in the redox reactions required for ATP production and it has been proposed that the energy failure due to ATP depletion which results from co-enzyme deficiency underlies the pathophysiology of the symptoms of pellagra [21]. As a result, it is the tissues with the highest turnover rates, such as the skin and mucous membranes, or organs with the highest energy demands, such as the brain, which are primarily affected by this nutritional deficiency disease. In addition to the redox reactions described above, NAD is also involved in other cellular processes, such as cell signalling and DNA repair. For example, NAD molecules are required for the formation of the PARP proteins which are involved in DNA repair and apoptosis [22]. Since the skin has a high cell turnover rate it is very susceptible to DNA damage during replication. This is particularly the case in sun-exposed areas of skin which are subject to solar radiation, where the NAD deficiency impairs the ability to repair the solar damage [23].

In terms of CNS functioning, there are thought to be a number of mechanisms whereby niacin deficiency can lead to the abnormalities observed in patients with pellagra. Firstly, 5-HT metabolism can be altered in patients with decreased niacin intake, since tryptophan can be shunted away from 5-HT synthesis to niacin production, in an attempt to restore physiological niacin levels [24]. The subsequent 5-HT deficiency which can result in pellagra patients may explain many of the CNS symptoms. Secondly, the tryptophan shunting will also decrease levels of another of its natural metabolites, kynurenic acid (KA). KA acts by inhibiting glutamate activity at the NMDA receptor [25], so the reduced synthesis which may result from niacin deficiency could lead to potentiation of the response to glutamate at the NMDA receptor. This could also be responsible for many of the CNS symptoms observed. Furthermore, KA deficiency has also been shown to reduce neurotoxicity thresholds in animal models [26], and may be responsible for the chromatolysis of neurones that can be seen in advanced stages of pellagra [27].

Psychiatric Aspects

The most widely reported CNS manifestation of the disease is its impact on cognitive functioning. All types of dementia are described in patients with pellagra, particularly in the later stages of the disease and in reference to the classical diagnostic triad. However, pellagra is probably better characterised by delirium rather than dementia, since the confused states described are similar to those seen in intoxication, are reversible with appropriate treatment and are found in association with electroencephalographic (EEG) evidence of diffuse slowing which is the hallmark sign of delirium [28 29]. A review of two of the first large scale American studies of the neuropsychological and behavioural aspects of pellagra in 1913 by Green [30] and 1915 by Singer31 indicated that the delirium often has an acute onset and is commonly accompanied by a lack of judgement and insight [32]. Patients become inattentive, disorientated in time and place and patients may be unable to perceive many everyday sensory stimuli such as movements in the visual field or tactile stimulation. This inability to focus attention may subsequently affect the ability to problem solve, evidenced by a number of pellagra patients reported to experience dyscalculia. Periods of memory loss, poor retention and the inability to recall basic school knowledge may also be experienced. The level of confusion may also fluctuate throughout the day, with episodes of severe confusion interspersed with episodes of clear thought [33] In the study by Green, the psychiatric diagnoses, demographic characteristics and results of neurological assessment were obtained for 131 patients with pellagra admitted to the Georgia State Sanitarium over a 20 month period (mean age = 37, range = 16-69) [30]. The average duration of psychiatric illness was 7 months, although this varied from 7 days to 8 years, and was generally shorter than the duration of other symptoms of pellagra (average duration = 11 months, range = 5 weeks to 8 years). Over half of the patients were classed as having an "infective-exhaustive psychosis", a term used to describe what would now be classified as delirium.

Although infrequently described in the pellagra literature, a number of neuropsychiatric symptoms other than delirium may present at any stage of the disease. These include hallucinations, disturbances of thought and delusional beliefs, as well as anxiety, depression and mania. A number of personality changes have also been reported which can lead to social isolation, violence and aggression [34]. In the patients studied by Green who were admitted to Georgia State Sanitarium, a manic-depressive psychosis was described in 12% of patients, whilst 11% were said to have "dementia praecox", disturbances in cognition that would now be classified as schizophrenia. Symptoms of depression and anxiety were also common, with 41% classed as having "depression" and 42% "apprehensiveness" [30]. In 1915 Singer analysed data from patients with pellagra from a larger population base, including patients seen in the community and in general hospitals in South Carolina and Georgia States [31]. The case records of 130 patients selected solely due to a positive diagnosis of pellagra demonstrated that psychiatric symptoms were present in 40.0%. It was also shown that as the number of attacks of pellagra increased, the frequency of psychiatric symptoms also increased and that the proportion of patients who subsequently died was significantly higher in patients who have psychiatric symptoms compared to those who do not (19.2% and 2.6%, respectively, $p<0.003$, FET), indicating that psychiatric symptoms present in more serious cases of the disease. Furthermore, mental illness was shown to be approximately 75 times more prevalent in patients with pellagra compared to the general population. The most common psychiatric diagnosis was depression, occurring in 31.5% of patients with the symptoms generally running a parallel clinical course to other symptoms of pellagra. Other psychiatric diagnoses were less common.

In a more recent study, the neuropsychiatric profiles of 20 consecutive patients with pellagra associated with chronic alcoholism were obtained from hospital records of patients admitted to the Kurate Kyoritsu Hospital in Miyatacho, Japan between 1965 and 1979 [27]. All of these patients were confused, 94.7% had hallucinations and 94.1% insomnia. Anxiety and depression were also observed in up to half of individuals. In addition to the above psychiatric symptoms observed in patients with pellagra, a number of extrapyramidal symptoms may also be present. One such symptom is paratonic rigidity, whereby there is involuntary resistance during passive movement proportional to the speed of the movement [35 36]. Other symptoms include *ante litteram* Parkinsonian features such as a festinating gait and tremor. These Parkinsonian features have been identified since the earliest descriptions of pellagra, with reports of patients with a "running disturbance of the limbs" as early as 1763 [37].

Whilst the majority of authors agree that the neuropsychiatric symptoms, especially the hallmark cognitive impairment, appear at later stages in the disease after the dermatological and gastrointestinal symptoms, Hoffer has argued that earliest pellagra symptoms may be anxiety, depression and fatigue, even in subclinical forms of pellagra [38]. This notion is supported by a number studies have demonstrated that pellagra should be suspected even if the hallmark dermatological or gastrointestinal signs and symptoms are not present [27 39]. It may also be of interest to note that self neglecting behaviours can also be present in patients with pellagra, especially those experiencing symptoms similar to a frontotemporal dementia. Resultantly, this could mean that patients fail to present with their symptoms until their disease has progressed to the late stages [40]. So far we have seen how neuropsychiatric illness can be a result of pellagra, but we must also examine how the nutritional deficiency responsible for pellagra can be caused by mental illness.

Firstly, some patients with chronic alcohol-dependence attain the majority of their dietary calories from alcohol and subsequently suffer from a number of nutritional deficiencies. In other patients with chronic alcohol-dependence without decreased dietary intake of niacin, pellagra can still be present. This is because alcohol damage to duodenal villi and other indirect results of alcohol damage can lead to decreased nutrient absorption [41]. Secondly, pellagra can be seen in the context of anorexia nervosa, with the dermatological features of the disease the most important diagnostic indicator in this population [14]. When treating patients with pellagra with nicotinamide, the dermatological and gastrointestinal symptoms usually resolve within 2 days and act as confirmation of a correct diagnosis. However, the neuropsychological symptoms respond in a less predictable manner, at one extreme taking a number of days and at the other persisting and leaving the patient with long term neuropsychological deficits [28].

CONCLUSION

In today's world, widespread vitamin supplementation and dietary education mean that the majority of individuals meet their daily niacin requirements. This is in stark contrast to the early 20th century, where pellagra rose to endemic levels and was one of the top 10 most common causes for mortality in America. The discovery that niacin deficiency was to blame lead to the introduction of food fortification programmes and successful treatments, and was therefore responsible for the declining prevalence throughout the rest of the century. Despite this, cases of pellagra are not rare in developing countries and may be on the increase in the developed world following immigration waves and possible increases in patients living with diseases including anorexia, HIV and alcohol-dependence. It is important to consider the full neuropsychiatric spectrum of pellagra, particularly since a number of patients may present with a clinical picture which does not exactly match the 'classical' diagnostic triad. Many of the above symptoms, such as depression and confusion can be seen in dementias. It is therefore suggested physicians maintain a high level suspicion for pellagra in patients who present with these symptoms and a history indicative of nutritional deficiency, even if the classical dermatological and gastrointestinal features are not present (e.g. *pellagra sine pellagra).*

REFERENCES

[1] Casal J. Historia natural, y médica de el Principado de Asturias. Madrid: Manuel Martín, 1762.

[2] Mariani-Costantini R, Mariani-Costantini A. An outline of the history of pellagra in Italy. *Journal of Anthropological Sciences* 2007;85:163-71.

[3] Dekleine W. Control of pellagra. *Southern Medical Journal* 1942;35(11).

[4] Bollet AJ. Politics and pellagra: the epidemic of pellagra in the U.S. in the early twentieth century. *Yale Journal of Biology and Medicine* 1992;65(3):211-21.

[5] Goldberger J. The etiology of pellagra. The significance of certain epidemiological observations with respect thereto. *Public Health Reports* 1914;29(26).

[6] Goldberger J, Wariu CH, Willets DG. The prevention of pellagra. A test of diet among institutional inmates. *Nutrition Reviews* 1973;31(5):152-53.

[7] Goldberger J, Wheeler GA, Lillie RD, Rogers LM. A further study of butter, fresh beef, and yeast as pellagra preventives, with consideration of the relation of factor P-P of pellagra (and black tongue of dogs) to vitamin B. *Public Health Reports* 1926;41(8):297-318.

[8] Elvehjem CA, Madden RJ, Strong FM, Woolley DW. Relation of nicotinic acid and nicotinic acid amide to canine black tongue. Journal of the American *Chemical Society* 1937;59(9):1767-68.

[9] Rajakumar K. Pellagra in the United States: a historical perspective. *Southern Medical Journal* 2000;93(3):272-7.

[10] Park YK, Sempos CT, Barton CN, Vanderveen JE, Yetley EA. Effectiveness of food fortification in the United States: the case of pellagra. *American Journal of Public Health* 2000;90(5):727-38.

[11] Pellagra and its prevention and control in major emergencies: *World Health Organisation,* 2000.

[12] Kertesz SG. Pellagra in 2 homeless men. *Mayo Clinic Proceedings* 2001;76(3):315-18.

[13] Cook CC, Hallwood PM, Thomson AD. B Vitamin deficiency and neuropsychiatric syndromes in alcohol misuse. *Alcohol and Alcoholism* 1998;33(4):317-36.

[14] Prousky JE. Pellagra may be a rare secondary complication of anorexia nervosa: a systematic review of the literature. *Alternative Medicine Review* 2003;8(2):180-5.

[15] Murray MF. Niacin as a potential AIDS preventive factor. *Medical Hypotheses* 1999;53(5):375-79.

[16] Bell HK, Poston GJ, Vora J, Wilson NJ. Cutaneous manifestations of the malignant carcinoid syndrome. *British Journal of Dermatology* 2005;152(1):71-5.

[17] Meyrick Thomas RH, Rowland Payne CM, Black MM. Isoniazid-induced pellagra. *British Medical Journal* 1981;283(6286):287-8.

[18] Stevens HP, Ostlere LS, Begent RH, Dooley JS, Rustin MH. Pellagra secondary to 5-fluorouracil. *British Journal of Dermatology* 1993;128(5):578-80.

[19] Karthikeyan K, Thappa DM. Pellagra and skin. *International Journal of Dermatology* 2002;41(8):476-81.

[20] Taori G, V. I. Neurological manifestations in nutritional deficiencies. In: Chopra JS, Arjundas G, Prabhakar S, eds. Textbook of Neurology. New Delhi: B.I. Churchill Livingston, 2001.

[21] Williams AC, Ramsden DB. Pellagra: A clue as to why energy failure causes diseases? *Med. Hypotheses* 2007;69(3):618-28.

[22] Oliver FJ, Menissier-de Murcia J, de Murcia G. Poly(ADP-ribose) polymerase in the cellular response to DNA damage, apoptosis, and disease. *American Journal of Human Genetics* 1999;64(5):1282-8.

[23] Brown TM. Pellagra: an old enemy of timeless importance. *Psychosomatics* 2010;51(2):93-7.

[24] Williams AC, Ramsden DB. Pellagra: A clue as to why energy failure causes diseases? *Medical Hypotheses* 2007;69(3):618-28.

[25] Elmslie KS, Yoshikami D. Effects of kynurenate on root potentials evoked by synaptic activity and amino acids in the frog spinal cord. *Brain Research* 1985;330(2):265-72.

[26] Poeggeler B, Rassoulpour A, Wu HQ, Guidetti P, Roberts RC, Schwarcz R. Dopamine receptor activation reveals a novel, kynurenate-sensitive component of striatal N-methyl-D-aspartate neurotoxicity. *Neuroscience* 2007;148(1):188-97.

[27] Ishii N, Nishihara Y. Pellagra among chronic alcoholics: clinical and pathological study of 20 necropsy cases. *Journal of Neurology, Neurosurgery and Psychiatry* 1981;44(3):209-15.

[28] Oldham M, Ivkovic A. Pellagrous encephalopathy presenting as alcohol withdrawal delirium: A case series and literature review. *Addiction Science and Clinical Practice* 2012;7(1):12.

[29] Sidhu KS, Balon R, Ajluni V, Boutros NN. Standard EEG and the difficult-to-assess mental status. *Annals of Clinical Psychiatry* 2009;21(2):103-8.

[30] Green BEM. A Review of 131 Cases of Pellagra. *Southern Medical Journal* 1913;6(3):171-73.

[31] Singer H. Mental and nervous disorders associated with pellagra. *Archives of Internal Medicine* 1915;XV(1):121-46.

[32] Williams A. How was cognition affected in cases of pellagra? *Parkinsonism and Related Disorders* 2009;15:S35-6.

[33] Lorenz WF. Mental Manifestations of Pellagra. *Public Health Reports* (1896-1970) 1916;31(5):221-46.

[34] Brozek J, Guetzkow H, Keys A. A study of personality of normal young men maintained on restricted intakes of vitamins of the B complex. *Psychosomatic Medicine* 1946;8:98-109.

[35] Serdaru M, Hausser-Hauw C, Laplane D, Buge A, Castaigne P, Goulon M, et al. The clinical spectrum of alcoholic pellagra encephalopathy. *Brain* 1988;111(4):829-42.

[36] Hobbelen JS, Koopmans RT, Verhey FR, Van Peppen RP, de Bie RA. Paratonia: a Delphi procedure for consensus definition. *Journal of Geriatric Physical Therapy* 2006;29(2):50-6.

[37] Cavanna AE, Williams AC. Neuropsychiatric symptoms in an early description of pellagra. *Journal of Neuropsychiatry and Clinical Neurosciences* 2010;22(4):E39.

[38] Hoffer A. Vitain B-3 dependency: chronic pellagra. *Townsend Letter for Doctors and Patients* 2000;207:66-73.

[39] Teare JP, Hyams G, Pollock S. Acute encephalopathy due to coexistent nicotinic acid and thiamine deficiency. *The British Journal of Clinical Practice* 1993;47(6):343-4.

[40] Amanullah S, Seeber C. Niacin deficiency resulting in neuropsychiatric symptoms: a case study and review of the literature. *Clinical Neuropsychiatry* 2010;7(1):10-14.

[41] Feinman L. Absorption and utilization of nutrients in alcoholism. *Alcohol Health and Research World* 1989;13(3):207-10.

INDEX

E

F

G

H

I

J

L

M

N

O

P

Q

R

S

T

U

V

W

Y